Understanding Dyslexia

Kathleen Anne Hennigh, M.A.

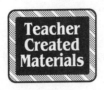
Teacher Created Materials

Teacher Created Materials, Inc.

Cover Design by Darlene Spivak

Made in U.S.A.
ISBN 1-55734-848-0
Order Number TCM 848

Table of Contents

Introduction

On March 1st, 1976, as a seven year old girl, I was diagnosed as dyslexic through the use of the Slingerland Screening Test for Identifying Children with Specific Language Disability. I showed the typical symptoms of dyslexia: consistent patterns of letter and word reversals, letter and word omissions, trouble memorizing, recalling, or identifying letters and words, and difficulty perceiving meaning in the letters and words. From that point on, afternoons were spent at a learning disability center or with a tutor. Unfortunately, in the classroom I continued to receive reading instruction through basal reading programs and was placed in low-ability reading groups. Most of my reading time was spent doing Silent Reading Activity (SRA). The SRA system has stories on several color coded cards, with each color designating a different ability level. Upon answering all questions correctly on one card, the student moves to the next color. I read slowly and rarely moved up in the color code. This experience left me feeling frustrated and unmotivated. On the outside I was always a dynamic person, quite able to communicate orally. But inside, I struggled with the belief that I was unintelligent.

The dyslexia label carries an acute stigma of mental incompetence. I was fortunate to have had parents who guided and believed in me, averting this stigma. However, many children with dyslexia do not have this support. Dyslexic children need to receive support from both parents and teachers.

This book is intended to give educators and parents a frame of reference regarding the topic of dyslexia. It provides practical methods of classroom instruction and home involvement which deal with the child's dyslexic reading patterns. Chapter one attempts to answer the question "What is dyslexia?" Chapter two explains the historical development of the word dyslexia. The third chapter outlines ideas for parental involvement in the home and school. Chapter four addresses the role of the teacher in the classroom. Chapter five discusses fundamental reading skills, while chapter six suggests methods for teaching language arts. The seventh chapter discusses how dyslexic patterns appear in other subject areas. Chapter eight provides methods for group work in the classroom. The book concludes with a methodology of assessing the performance and progression of dyslexic students. I sincerely hope this book is useful to you.

Dyslexia

What Is Dyslexia?

The Webster dictionary defines dyslexia as a disturbance of the ability to read (Webster, 1987). However, diagnosing dyslexia is not that simple. At some point in our lives, we have all probably had difficulty with reading to a certain degree. In addition, the term "dyslexic" has been misused and overused in the past twenty years. Dyslexia is characterized by a consistent difficulty with processing phonological information. A phoneme is the smallest unit of speech sound. Processing phonological information refers to the identification, pronunciation, and use of the different speech sounds in language. Typical dyslexic patterns involve:

♦ Reversing letters in reading and writing

♦ Omitting words in reading and writing

♦ Difficulty converting letters into sounds and words

♦ Difficulty using sounds to create words

♦ Difficulty recalling sounds and letters from memory

♦ Difficulty perceiving meaning from letters and words

> Dyslexia is characterized by a consistent difficulty with processing phonological information.

It is important to realize that everyone exhibits these patterns at some time during reading development. Dyslexia refers to the condition a child has when these patterns occur consistently and repeatedly.

Dyslexia as a Learning Disability

The conditions described as dyslexia have frequently been referred to as a "learning disability." The learning disability view sees dyslexia as a subcategory of learning disorders which pertains to reading (Mayo Clinic, 1993). This may lead to much confusion. People often use the term dyslexia to refer to learning disorders in general, rather than to the specific reading deficiency.

The learning disability view also focuses on a child's inability to recognize letters and words on the printed page. However, the distinguishing criteria is a comparison to peers. If the child is reading at an ability level below the expected level for the age of that child, he or she can be seen to have a reading disability. It is when the lower ability level is a product of the child's difficulty recognizing letters and words that the term dyslexia is used.

Although most definitions of dyslexia acknowledge a type of severe reading pattern, there is no single clear conception of the cause.

Causes of Dyslexia

There is much debate over the cause of dyslexia. Like a learning disability, dyslexia is a condition that everyone seems to agree exists, but about which there is little agreement otherwise (Gillet & Temple, 1990). Although most definitions of dyslexia acknowledge a type of severe reading pattern, there is no single clear conception of the cause. The most widespread belief is that dyslexia is a neurological disorder, characterized by frequent letter and word reversals (Orton, 1937).

Although the basis of dyslexia is unknown, there is evidence that it is caused by a malfunction of certain areas of the brain concerned with language (Mayo Clinic, 1993). Dr. Albert Galaburda of Harvard University Medical School found that brain cells of dyslexic people are organized in unusual ways and have a different structure than a nondyslexic brain (Jones, 1992). Test results have indicated that brains of deceased dyslexics, when compared to brains of nondyslexics, had different organization of nerve cells. The dyslexic brains were found to have significantly more misplaced and unusually organized nerve cells, especially in the language regions (Flowers, 1993). Further tests showed that the neural tissue present in the dyslexics' temporal planum, a section of the brain that deals with linguistics, was larger in the right hemisphere. In the general population, this region is usually larger in the left hemisphere (Flowers, 1993).

Additionally, a family history of reading difficulties is often found when investigating the dyslexic person's genetic heritage (Mayo Clinic, 1993).

An argument can be made, however, that dyslexia is truly a characterization of defective reading patterns which may be more environmentally induced than neurologically mandated. In this situation, each child needs to be looked at individually in order to try to pinpoint the environmental cause. In some instances, family problems, divorce, neglect, or abuse can be the cause of the reading difficulty. The most frustrating aspect in the assessment of dyslexia is that there seems to be no single underlying cause (Rayner & Pollatsek, 1989).

Diagnosis in the Classroom

Whatever the reason may be that a person shows dyslexic reading patterns, the pragmatic teacher should not focus on the cause but rather the patterns. It is important to note that the teacher does not diagnose the child for dyslexia or any learning disability. A learning disability should be diagnosed by a trained reading or language specialist. However, the teacher is most often the first to detect a possible reading problem or learning disability and is the first step in referring a child for further testing.

Dyslexia is a consistency of these reading patterns: reversals, omissions, and difficulty using sounds, letters and words. To detect dyslexia in the classroom, teachers need to be keen observers and be aware of how their students read. The first step every teacher can take if he or she suspects possible dyslexic reading patterns is to administer informal reading tests. Informal reading tests do not require training to administer, and the classroom teacher may conduct them. Two tests that are easy to give and reveal much information about the child's reading habits are a Qualitative Reading Inventory and a Running Record.

Qualitative Reading Inventory (QRI)

A Qualitative Reading Inventory (Leslie & Caldwell, 1990) is a preprinted, commercial assessment tool that allows a teacher, with little preparation, to assess a child's reading ability. The QRI consists of grade level word lists with stories corresponding to each list. First the child reads the word lists. Then, the teacher selects the story corresponding to the list the child read at 90% accuracy. Next, the child's prior knowledge on the story's topic is activated. The teacher asks questions prior to reading the story about the upcoming subject matter. If the story is about a certain animal, does the child

The first step every teacher can take if he or she suspects possible dyslexic reading patterns is to administer informal reading tests.

3

know anything about that animal? If the child is unfamiliar with that animal, that may affect his or her comprehension. In this case, the teacher can select another story. The child then reads the selected story aloud. As the child reads, the teacher has a copy of the text and marks words the child reads automatically, words the child must decode or sound out, and words the child omits, repeats, or substitutes. After the passage is read, the teacher asks the child to retell the story in his or her own words.

Finally, four or five questions are asked about the text to check for comprehension. All answers are recorded verbatim in the child's words. The major purpose of the QRI is to provide a profile of the strengths and weaknesses of a child's reading, word recognition, strategies used when dealing with an unfamiliar word, reading patterns, and comprehension. To identify a child who possibly is dyslexic, the teacher can compare the child's highest instructional level with his or her grade placement. The teacher should also observe the reading patterns and look for consistent reversals, omissions, and difficulty with sounds, letters, and word recognition. If there is consistency, then the teacher can refer the child for testing.

To identify a child who possibly is dyslexic, the teacher can compare the child's highest instructional level with his or her grade placement.

Running Record

Instead of using the QRI, a teacher can assess the child's reading patterns using a running record (Clay, 1979). The running record method is similar to the QRI in having the child read a selected text aloud while the teacher marks on his or her own copy of the text exactly what the child reads. The difference is that the running record method can be used without purchasing the QRI's commercial material. However, this requires more preparation by the teacher.

The method is as follows: The teacher first selects a story. The text used should be interesting to the child and should be at his or her instructional level (within a 90% accuracy). Then, the child reads the story. Just as with the QRI, the teacher notes each reading mistake. Teachers should record when the child shows consistent patterns such as:

◆ Stuttering

◆ Repeating a word or phrase

◆ Substituting a word

◆ Reversing words

◆ Mispronouncing words

◆ Omitting a word

◆ Self-correction

As the teacher reads along with the child, the teacher makes marks after each word. Checks can be placed on top of words that are read correctly. Special notations or codes can be placed above each inaccurately read word, designating the type of mistake. After the child reads the text, the teacher can ask comprehension questions. However, certain questions should be avoided:

◆ Avoid long or complicated questions. The child may spend more time interpreting the question than giving an answer, and it is difficult to evaluate which thought process presents more of a problem for the child, the question or the answer.

◆ Avoid yes or no questions. These questions are usually not useful in testing a child's comprehension, since there is automatically a 50% chance of accuracy.

◆ Avoid questions that can be answered without reading the text.

◆ Avoid asking questions geared at memorization of lists involved in the story's plot (e.g., "What things did the main characters do when they woke up in the morning?"), rather than questions which challenge the child to interpret the plot (Vacca, Vacca, & Gove, 1991).

If consistent dyslexic reading patterns are observed, the teacher can refer the child for testing with a reading or language specialist.

After the running record is administered, teachers should analyze the results by looking for consistent dyslexic reading patterns. Teachers can compare the story level the child read with 90% accuracy with his or her own grade leve!. Most importantly teachers should look for the dyslexic reading patterns. A running record can be administered daily or weekly and each test can be compared to the others to check for consistency. If consistent dyslexic reading patterns are observed, the teacher can refer the child for testing with a reading or language specialist.

Whether the teacher uses a QRI or a running record, much information can be gained that will help the teacher decide whether the child needs to be referred for further diagnosis and testing for a reading disability. If the child clearly exhibits dyslexic reading patterns, then a specialist should analyze the process and quality of the child's reading skills. The specialized testing will be conducted with greater ease if the teacher keeps dated, specific observations and if reading assessments have already been administered.

Another step the teacher can take in diagnosing a child is to investigate the medical and family history. Teachers should check the child's background files for vision, hearing, or nutritional problems. The reading difficulty may be the result of vision or hearing impairment. Visual, hearing, and neurological tests should be given to verify that the child's difficulty is not due to another disorder (Mayo Clinic, 1993). In addition, the dyslexic reading patterns might be the result of problems at home or malnutrition. If the child is not eating correctly, teachers can keep track of his or her eating habits and make note of how that affects learning in the classroom. If teachers discover a family problem, such as divorce or a death in the family, it is possible that the child may be referred to counseling. The teacher can then see if the child's learning improves in the classroom while he or she receives counseling. Even if a divorce in the family or malnutrition is not the cause of the reading difficulty, the teacher is dealing with problems in the child's life and addressing them in a positive way. Whether the teacher can pinpoint the cause of the reading difficulty or not, the important thing is to try to find ways to compensate for it or eliminate it.

Concluding Remarks

The above issues are the most difficult areas of dyslexia, the definition, the cause, and the diagnosis. The best thing a teacher in the classroom can do is to be aware of his or her students. Teachers should observe the students and look for consistent dyslexic reading patterns. Teachers should know their students' medical and family backgrounds. If there is any suspicion of a learning disability, teachers can administer informal reading tests and refer students for further testing. Regardless of whether a child is diagnosed as dyslexic, the methods discussed in this book will help children who have difficulty with reading as well as the rest of the children in the classroom.

Whether the teacher can pinpoint the cause of the reading difficulty or not, the important thing is to try to find ways to compensate for it or eliminate it.

History of Dyslexia

Definition of the Term

Teachers who educate themselves with background knowledge on dyslexia and other learning disabilities will have an easier time understanding the problem. It is with that goal that I add this chapter on the history of dyslexia.

Difficulty with reading and writing was first characterized only as an aphasia.

Since the term "dyslexia" was first used in 1887, researchers have had difficulty defining it (Ekwall & Shanker, 1983). Simplistically, the Latin "dys" means "bad or difficult," and the Greek root "lexia" means "read" so dyslexia means "difficulty with reading."

Aphasia

Difficulty with reading and writing was first characterized only as an aphasia. The term aphasia means loss or impairment of the ability to use or comprehend words due to an injury to the brain. The term has been with us since the early 19th century. Neurologists describe four different kinds of aphasia. First, we have sensory aphasia which is difficulty understanding spoken language. Second, motor aphasia, which is difficulty expressing thoughts. Third, alexia, which is difficulty reading. Finally, agraphia, which is difficulty with writing. When the term dyslexia was introduced, it was classified generally as one of the aphasias, usually alexia (Richardson, 1992).

Word Blindness

In 1877, Adolph Kussmaul came up with the term "word blindness." Although still referring to a product of brain injury, this terminology further delineated the condition we now know as dyslexia. Word blindness describes the situation where an individual's capacity for sight, speech, and intelligence are intact, but there is an inability of the patient to recognize words that the patient already knows. In 1892, J. Dejerine stated that word blindness was due to a lesion in the angular gyrus of the brain (Richardson, 1989). The angular gyrus is a part of the brain that deals with language. He later added that such a lesion would produce agraphia. The first child to have been reported with congenital word blindness was in 1896 by Dr. W. Pringle Morgan, a physician, in Sussex, England.

Dyslexia

Dr. Rudolf Berlin first introduced the term dyslexia in 1887 (Richardson, 1989). Dyslexia was seen as an acquired condition, developed after birth. However, Berlin suggested this difficulty with reading may be due to "cerebral disease" rather than a brain injury. Dyslexia was seen as "describing a special group of patients who experienced great difficulty in reading because of cerebral disease" (Richardson, 1989, p. 7). Significantly, Berlin's analysis appears to be the first recognition that dyslexic reading patterns can occur without a severe trauma to the head.

Scottish ophthalmologist J. Hinshelwood in his book *Congenital Word Blindness* (1917) observed that there were often several cases in one family. Symptoms paralleled those appearing in the adults who had lost the capacity to read because of injury to the brain (Richardson, 1989). Hinshelwood stated that the reading difficulty might come from underdevelopment of the angular gyrus rather than merely a lesion. His work was conducted mainly on postmortem analyses of subjects, and he felt that the brain underdevelopment might also be due to disease, birth injury, or genetic disposition (Hinshelwood, 1917; Richardson, 1989). Hinshelwood believed that the dyslexic patterns could be alleviated through one-on-one teaching and use of multisensory approaches. By stimulating more than one cerebral center (sight, smell, touch, taste) the subject would have more means of interpretation.

> Significantly, Berlin's analysis appears to be the first recognition that dyslexic reading patterns can occur without a severe trauma to the head.

Samuel Orton is generally regarded as the foremost researcher of dyslexia. In 1928 he described the condition of reversals in reading as strephosymbolia, which means "twisted symbols." Although the terminology never caught on, the idea is now commonly seen as the same problem of reversals described in dyslexia. Orton put forth the mixed dominance theory that dyslexia was caused by poorly established dominance of one side of the brain over the other. When a person would view a symbol, the right and left sides of the brain would each independently encode the symbol. Each side's encoded version was a reversed, mirror image of the other. Confusion came from there being a lack of one side of the brain's established dominance over the other side. Until such dominance was established, there would be uncertainty over which mirror image to follow, and thus the problem of reversals would continue.

Orton did not view dyslexia as stemming from a brain injury or defect. Although he saw the problem of dyslexia as largely physiological, he viewed it as a developmental problem and not entirely congenital. Dyslexia may be said to include both the hereditary tendency and the environmental forces which are brought to play on the individual (Orton, 1937). The developmental focus centered on the delay a dyslexic child had in acquiring language. Children who were dyslexic demonstrated a reading ability much below the expected level for their ages. Importantly, Orton did not view each of the children's language skills (reading, writing, speaking, listening) independently. He focused on the unitary nature of the language system and emphasized that a delay in acquiring reading skills could be a delay in the development of the entire system devoted to language (Orton, 1937; Richardson, 1989). However, some dyslexic children have an easier time communicating orally than they do communicating in writing.

Samuel Orton is generally regarded as the foremost researcher of dyslexia.

Over the years the term dyslexia has come to mean so many different things to people that one may argue the word has limited value today. Many people simply use the term "learning disabled" for children with any language difficulty or slowness in development, adding the specifics of individual conditions accordingly (Ekwall & Shanker, 1983). Often parents will describe their child as learning disabled or "L.D." and then continue to describe the child's difficulty with transposing characters while reading.

Functional Definitions

Many researchers and teachers feel that the traditional method of defining dyslexia according to what it is not is no longer useful in diagnosing the child's real situation. For purposes of this book, the issue will be illustrated so that teachers and parents may expand their understanding of dyslexia and decide upon a definition that is most helpful.

Exclusionary Definition

Traditionally, dyslexic children have been identified by the use of exclusionary criteria. The World Federation definition describes dyslexia in general as a difficulty learning to read. It then proceeds to exclude other characteristics which are not within the definition, such as low intelligence and socio-cultural background. The definition suggested by the World Federation of Neurology (1968; cited in Kamhi, 1992, p. 49) is:

> *Specific developmental dyslexia is a disorder manifested by difficulty learning to read, despite conventional instruction, adequate intelligence, and socio-cultural opportunity. It is dependent upon fundamental cognitive disabilities which are frequently of constitutional origin.*

The exclusionary definition is often applied with the stipulation that the child has normal intelligence but reads two grades below the level of his or her peers.

Many argue that the exclusionary definition is not useful because it provides a very limited description of the disorder's characteristics. Instead of describing specific characteristics to search for, the definition merely directs us to look for a general difficulty in learning to read and then eliminate other possible causes. Additionally, since the definition's only hallmark is "difficulty learning to read," the child must first experience some degree of failure before he or she can fall within the definition (Kamhi, 1992). The definition neglects to recognize that a dyslexic pattern of language learning may be discovered before the child actually learns to read. With any type of language learning, there is an obvious need for early identification of problems since the formative years of a child are so important to literacy growth. When difficulty acquiring language is identified early on, then the difficulty can be compensated for with strategic learning or, hopefully, eliminated before dyslexic reading patterns are manifested.

The exclusionary definition is often applied with the stipulation that the child has normal intelligence but reads two grades below the level of his or her peers. How can one determine if a child in first grade is reading below two grade levels? Often the disparity of a child reading two grade levels below his or her peers cannot be established until the third grade (Jones, 1992). This presents an additional obstacle to early detection, since the child in kindergarten or first grade cannot be relatively compared. In addition, in light of the popularity of multi-age classrooms, there is a fundamental question of whether to use grade levels at all since children may learn at different rates.

Inclusionary Definition

In contrast to the exclusionary definition is the inclusionary definition which delimits the specific abilities and disabilities that characterize individuals with dyslexia (Kamhi, 1992). Inclusionary definitions focus on identifying the nature of language itself and isolating the difficulty dyslexics have in processing phonological information. While the exclusionary definition has been used for a long time, the inclusionary definition seems to be more in vogue with current thinking. The definition stated below is advocated by Alan Kamhi (1992):

> *Dyslexia is a developmental language disorder whose defining characteristic is a life-long difficulty processing phonological information. This difficulty involves encoding, retrieving, and using phonological codes in memory as well as deficits in phonological awareness and speech production. The disorder, which is often genetically transmitted, is generally present at birth and persists throughout the life span. A prominent characteristic of the disorder is spoken and written language deficiencies* (Kamhi, 1992, p. 50).

The essence of the inclusionary definition is to note that it can be difficult to distinguish between "poor" readers and children with dyslexia.

Kamhi discusses points which he believes may make this definition more adequate. First, it defines the disorder according to specific characteristics (encoding, retrieving, and phonological awareness) rather than simply stating it as a reading disability. Second, by specifying the nature of the phonological processing, the definition excludes individuals who may have reading problems due to other sources (hearing loss, visual or mental impairment). Third, the definition does not extend into other "domains of cognitive functioning" such as comprehension and reasoning (Kamhi, 1992). The essence of the inclusionary definition is to note that it can be difficult to distinguish between "poor" readers and children with dyslexia. This definition allows for the existence of a distinction.

The inclusionary definition also has drawbacks because it is geared toward being more specific. In some cases, depending on the definition, it may be too specific. For example, Kamhi's definition of dyslexia states that the condition must be "life long" and that it is "often genetically transmitted." The goal of an educator is to teach children to compensate for dyslexic reading patterns so that as adults the patterns are not displayed. Therefore, absent conclusive supporting research, defining dyslexia as "life long" may be too specific. Further, for practical purposes, a dyslexic reading pattern exists regardless of the cause. To suggest that the disorder is "often genetically transmitted" is a matter of continuing debate, and to incorporate this debate within the definition may be too specific for the practical purposes of correcting the disorder. Since an inclusionary definition is characteristically specific, it may force the educator to choose between definitions to find the one she or he believes is most accurate.

Proposed "Working" Definition

For the purpose of this book, the students that I believe need remediation are students who experience consistent frustration in learning how to process phonological information: identification, pronunciation, and use of the different speech sounds in language. This may affect all areas of language use: listening, speaking, reading, and writing. When given IQ tests, these children's scores reveal normal or even high intelligence. These dyslexic reading patterns are not due to brain injury, second language acquisition, or a language dialect. While children whose primary language is not English can display dyslexic reading patterns, these patterns are due to the natural challenges of learning English.

These dyslexic reading patterns are not due to brain injury, second language acquisition, or a language dialect.

Concluding Remarks

The search for a specific definition and cause of dyslexia is ongoing. In order to avoid damage to the child's self-esteem, early identification is strongly encouraged as the child's suffering increases the longer he or she experiences failure. Finally, the focus of remediation should be on the student's abilities and strengths rather than the challenges and weaknesses. Much can be done to encourage compensation and the ability to "work around problems."

Parents of the
Dyslexic Child

Parent Support

It is important for the dyslexic child to have strong parental support. Teachers can discuss the following information and activities with parents of dyslexic students, since what happens at home can affect the child's life in school. When the parents and the teacher are working together in a consistent program to help the child learn, the child will experience success sooner. Some parents go into denial and will not admit or even discuss the possibility that their child has a learning disability. Other parents will have questions about dyslexia that are sometimes difficult for the teacher to answer. Hopefully this chapter will make an uncomfortable situation a little bit easier.

> Some parents go into denial and will not admit or even discuss the possibility that their child has a learning disability.

Observations Before the Child Enters School

Before the child even enters school, there are things that a parent can look for. Many times the parent is the first to be aware of difficulty. Since no two children are alike in genetic makeup, it is hard to specify characteristics of dyslexia, and we cannot assume that all

13

children will behave in the same way. Cronin (1994) discusses some things to look for early on. While parents can say that all children display these behaviors to some degree, the dyslexic child will display the characteristics more frequently and more severely.

- ◆ Mixed laterality; no preference for left or right hand
- ◆ Inability to follow a sequence of instructions
- ◆ Does not pay attention
- ◆ Cannot sit still
- ◆ Disturbs others
- ◆ Becomes irritable easily
- ◆ Stubborn
- ◆ Does not finish work
- ◆ Immature

Just because a child may not show motor skill or coordination right away does not mean these skills will not come later.

Again, no two children are alike and the observations are what parents should work with. Cronin (1994) discusses eight areas for the parents to observe:

- ◆ 1. *Motor skills*: Does the child cut well? Run well?
- ◆ 2. *Motor coordination:* Does the child color in the lines? Walk in a straight line? Throw a ball?
- ◆ 3. *Sense of space:* Does the child know left from right? Complete simple puzzles? Have a sense of time?
- ◆ 4. *Memory sequence:* Does the child follow two-step directions? Remember three-item lists?
- ◆ 5. *Language:* Does the child act out ideas rather then use words? Use limited vocabulary?
- ◆ 6. *Choices:* Does the child make independent choices?
- ◆ 7. *Social maturity:* Does the child socialize with others?
- ◆ 8. *Behavior:* Does the child show frustration easily?

Parents should make specific notes when observing their child. The form on the following page can be used to make observations. If parents are sensitive and aware of their child's behavior and growth pattern, then observations can be made in order to decide whether further actions should be taken. Child development occurs at many different speeds. Just because a child may not show motor skill or coordination right away does not mean these skills will not come later. The signs to look for are a continuous lack of these skills.

Parent Observation Form

Student's Name _____

Name of parent completing form: _____

Please place a check under the appropriate response.

	Usually	Sometimes	Rarely
Participates in family conversations			
Follows directions			
Enjoys being read to			
Understands basic plot			
Enjoys talking about books			
Checks out books from library			
Draws pictures for stories			
Uses conventional spelling			
Enjoys talking about writing			

Questions I have:

Comments:

Reprinted from TCM777 Language Arts Assessment, *Teacher Created Materials, 1994*

When a child is professionally diagnosed as dyslexic, one of the first reactions parents may have is that their child has an illness (Hartwig, 1984). Dyslexia is not an illness, but the emotions a family may experience are similar to the experience of having a family member with an illness. Leonard Hartwig (1984), the parent of a dyslexic child, discusses five stages that parents may go through after hearing that their child is a dyslexic:

◆ 1. *Denial:* "It must be a mistake, not my child."

◆ 2. *Anger:* "Why did this have to happen to me?"

◆ 3. *Depression:* "My child isn't normal."

◆ 4. *Acceptance:* "Accept the fact, get help, get involved."

◆ 5. *Hope:* "My child can and will learn."

So many times the focus lies on what the dyslexic child can not do rather than all of the child's abilities and talents.

Many parents may feel that getting to the hope stage is impossible, but a positive attitude is essential and the parent needs to express that hope to the child. Parents should recognize what their child can do and make a point of praising the child's abilities. So many times the focus lies on what the dyslexic child cannot do rather than all of the child's abilities and talents. Hartwig (1984) discusses some common sense guides for the parents of a dyslexic child:

◆ Do not be overprotective. Dyslexic children are very capable and should take on responsibility.

◆ Do not do for the child what he or she can do for him or herself. Give the child a chance to try things out.

◆ Encourage curiosity and special interests the child may have, such as art, music, or sports. Children are more motivated when it involves something they enjoy.

◆ Set reasonable goals but do not make things too easy or too difficult.

◆ Be patient. Becoming upset or anxious will only frustrate the child.

◆ Think long-term and view the future objectively. Dyslexic children should be encouraged to attend college and receive higher degrees.

Many times when a dyslexic child experiences frustration, parents are unaware of how that affects their expectations of the child. Dyslexic children can be highly intelligent and very capable. However, parents can react in a way that undermines the child's strengths and reinforces the weaknesses.

Many parents provide negative feedback when instructing the child on a problem-solving task, which lowers self-expectations and self-esteem. Parents of children with dyslexia may not ask questions but, rather, may tell their child the information. This kind of behavior maintains the child's low motivation and self-expectations which in turn connects to the child's learning problem (Lyytinen, Rasku–Puttonen, Poikkeus, Laakso, & Ahonen, 1994). Parents help children develop representational thinking by placing mental demands on the child to reconstruct events, anticipate possible outcomes, and attend to transformations. Parents should be aware of their questioning strategies. Questions that encourage deeper thinking will lead the child to higher levels of thinking. Children will begin to think operatively and search for solutions (Lyytinen, et al., 1994). The interaction between parents and a dyslexic child should allow the child to dominate and guide the learning experience. The child should be active rather than passive, which will lead to less dependence on the parent.

Parents who provide their child with a positive atmosphere of praise and encouragement will set an easier path for the child's growth. It is crucial that the child has support, encouragement and understanding from parents and that parents realize that remediation takes time (Huston, 1992). These expectations should be developed early on and the interaction between the parent and child should be one focused on positive learning, exploring, and growing.

Parents who provide their child with a positive atmosphere of praise and encouragement will set an easier path for the child's growth.

Reading and Vocabulary Activities

Often both parents work full time and have busy schedules. There are many activities that can take just 15–30 minutes a day which can make a big difference in a dyslexic child's life. The important thing to do is to try to establish a routine. Dyslexic children need structure and organization in their lives (Tuttle & Paquette, 1994). Parents should keep directions short and clear. The interaction should be nonthreatening and inviting for success. Parents can refer to the guide on the following page to help their child to read.

Parent's Guide
"Helping Your Child to Read"

1. Set a good example. Read for pleasure and show and share that pleasure.

2. Leave interesting books lying around. Encourage your child to handle books frequently, carefully, and respectfully.

3. Read aloud eagerly to your child. Show him or her how much you enjoy this reading time. Make it special and do it each night if possible.

4. Provide a good reading light for your child's bed area. Encourage a relaxing nightly reading period. Give your child a special hug as you turn off the light at bedtime.

5. Be tuned in to what interests your child. Find books and other reading material in these areas of interest.

6. Discuss books and current events as a family.

7. Ask your child to read to you. Don't be anxious or impatient with his or her reading ability. Listen to the child read; do not listen for reading mistakes.

8. Encourage your child to share what he or she has read in books. Discuss stories, plots, characters, conflicts, resolutions, and feelings.

9. Visit the library together. Be sure your child has a library card and encourage its use. Use yours, too!

10. Share a reading interest. Both of you read books on the same subject and share what you've learned.

11. Be pleased with your child's reading progress. Give specific and genuine praise.

Reprinted from TCM354 Literature Activities for Reluctant Readers, *Teacher Created Materials, 1991*

Reading Aloud

Some parents of learning disabled children think that the best way for their child to learn is with flash cards, spelling drills, and skills activities. These activities, although of some help, can be boring and develop very little motivation on the part of the child. One of the best things a parent can do for a child with dyslexic patterns is to read stories aloud to the child. At any age, we enjoy hearing a good story. In addition, children learn that books are important to the parent (Griffiths, 1978). Parents should pick stories about topics that interest the child. Stories can be short and take as little as 10 minutes. When a parent reads aloud to a child, he or she gives the child a positive experience with reading while, at the same time, modeling positive reading habits.

Vocabulary Box

Another activity that parents can do with children is to keep a vocabulary box. The word can be written on one side of a 3 x 5 (8 cm x 13 cm) card and the definition of the word on the opposite side. The child can decorate the outside of the box. Parents can ask their child questions like "Do you know what that sign says?" or "Do you know what that word means?" while driving in the car and then add new words to the vocabulary box. While at the table eating dinner, parents can use words in sentences and then ask the child if he or she knows what the word means. New words can be added regularly to the child's box. Eventually, the child will begin to ask what words mean when he or she hears something unfamiliar without the parent suggesting the words. Finally, once a week, the parent and child can go through the words in the box, spelling the words correctly and saying what the words mean. It is important to always start from the beginning of the box and go through all of the words each time. The repetition will help the child learn the words faster.

> One of the best things a parent can do for a child with dyslexic patterns is to read stories out loud to the child.

Daily Activities

A final activity that is extremely practical and useful is to incorporate reading in daily events. When parents are driving in the car with their child, they can have the child become aware of direction by pointing out when a left or right turn is made. Parents can point out buildings and ask the child if he or she knows which side of the street the building is on (Cronin, 1994). When at the store or market, parents can point out items they put in the basket and ask the child to identify the objects. When the child looks at a box of cereal and says the word cereal, parents can show the child where the word is written on the box. These simple activities increase print awareness. Plus, the child feels that he or she is able to read.

In addition, the dinner table can be a wonderful place for conversation and family discussion (Huston, 1992). Today, dinner is often spent in front of the television or with the television on in the background. Parents should turn off the television and ask their child about his or her day. Parents can ask the child not only about the positive things in the day but also about anything that may be troubling or frustrating. Parents should give positive reinforcement if the child brings up something that was exciting or rewarding.

Writing and Comprehension Activities

When working with the dyslexic child, many times the focus lies on skills and not meaning. Dyslexic children receive little training in reading comprehension with almost exclusive focus on decoding (Clark, 1988). Parents can engage in reading activities with their child that focus on higher levels of thinking in a positive, enjoyable way. These activities can take 15–30 minutes and can influence a child's self-esteem, success in the classroom, and the relationship between the child and parents.

> When working with the dyslexic child, many times the focus lies on skills and not meaning.

Bedtime Story

Again, an activity that can be quick and effective is a bedtime story. Many times a parent reads through the story with little interaction. Throughout the reading of the story the parent should be asking the child questions. To begin, the parent should show the cover of the book to the child and ask what he or she thinks the story will be about, what he or she sees on the cover, and what he or she thinks the title is about. Next, a parent should read through the first few pages and ask the child to tell what has happened so far in the story in his or her own words, who the characters are, where the story takes place, why the characters did what they did, and what will happen next. Finally, at the end of the story, the parent can ask what the story was about, why it ended the way it did, and what the child liked or disliked. Interaction should be informal and enjoyable.

Journals

Another activity that parents can encourage their child to do is keep a journal. In a journal the child can write down what was done during the day and record feelings about family, friends, and school. If the child is young and has difficulty writing, then pictures can be drawn about the day, what was done and feelings. The journal can be personal or shared, and the child should be told that spelling does not matter (Huston, 1992). However the child expresses him or herself, he or she is learning to put thoughts down on paper. Parents need to have a special time set aside for the child to work in the journal, which can be done for 15 minutes a night. This should not be a chore but encouraged as a pleasure. Parents can get their own journals and have journal time with their child, setting a good example.

Alphabet Letters

Finally, every child should have a set of alphabet letters that can help in spelling, writing, print awareness, and letter recognition. There are various types of letters that can be used. Parents can get large wooden letters that lay flat or stand up. There are also aluminum letters used for mailboxes that are smooth and cool (Griffiths, 1978). Another type of less expensive alphabet letters can be made out of cardboard. The right side of the letter should be bright, shiny, and colorful while the flip side of the letter should be covered with a dull gray color (Griffiths, 1978). Parents can spell out words for the child and then ask the child to pull out the letters. There should always be free playtime for the child to simply explore with the letters. Parents should encourage the child to spell out his or her name or favorite foods. Correcting the child if the word is misspelled should be done gently. Parents should never say, "that's wrong" or "you messed up." Negative comments like this are unmotivating and promote low self-esteem. Parents can simply say, "good try, you just need to add this letter" or "switch these letters and it's perfect."

Communication between the teacher and the parents of a dyslexic child is key to the learning process and the success of the child.

Parent and the Teacher

Communication between the teacher and the parents of a dyslexic child is key to the learning process and success of the child. A program that sets reasonable goals, ways to reach these goals, and ideas for follow-up should be set up with the child, parent, and teacher. Meetings should be set regularly so that the program can be monitored. While parents may have busy schedules and little time, they still need to meet with the teacher on a regular basis. Before the parent meets with the teacher for the first time, Cronin (1994) lists certain questions the parent should consider:

- ◆ Is my child organized?
- ◆ Does my child have a short attention span?
- ◆ Does my child forget things?
- ◆ Does my child daydream?
- ◆ Does my child distract easily?
- ◆ What strategies does my child have?
- ◆ How does my child learn best?
- ◆ What are my child's interests?
- ◆ What does my child like to do?

Parents should bring this information to the conference and share it with the teacher. The parent should also have a list of any questions he or she may have for the teacher. In addition, teachers should be prepared for the conference with observations, sample work, and questions about the child's home life.

There are many ways teachers and parents can communicate. First, teachers and parents can communicate by meeting together twice a month simply to review the child's progress and any changes that need to be made. Second, the parents and teacher can have a folder or notebook that can be sent back and forth with notes, questions, and comments written inside. The teacher can put the journal in the child's backpack when he or she leaves school and the parent can put the notebook in the backpack when the child leaves home in the morning. Soon the child will learn to be responsible and take the notebook back and forth on his or her own. The notebook will encourage constant communication even if the teacher simply writes "A good day!"

Children should always be involved with the goal setting meeting as well as the whole evaluation process.

In addition, goals need to be set up with the teacher, parents and child. The goals should be revised every two to three months and should be realistic. For example, the child can have three goals:

- ◆ 1. Read a book every day.
- ◆ 2. Write in my journal every day.
- ◆ 3. Raise my hand in class and participate in discussions.

These goals can be easily checked through the teacher and parent and are specific, concrete, and simple to understand. Using home reading logs and writing logs, the child can learn organizational skills while the parents keep track of how much the child is reading and writing at home (Ryan, 1994). Goals should be evaluated and changed once the child, teacher, and parents feel that the expectations have been met. Children should always be involved with the goal setting meeting as well as in the whole evaluation process. Children should understand why a goal needs to be worked on and how the goal can be achieved. This will develop independence, self-awareness, and self-evaluation.

Tutors and Homework

With many children growing up in single parent households or in homes where both parents work, there is often not enough time for a parent to work with his or her child on a regular basis. Through the use of a tutor, homework can become less of a burden and more of an enjoyable experience. The tutor can help the child develop strategies that will eventually help the child do the homework on his or her own. Many times a tutor can be a sibling, a sibling's friend, or an older student from school. There are certain guidelines Cronin (1994) discusses when doing homework with or without a tutor that can help the dyslexic child experience less frustration and more success.

- ◆ 1. Set up a routine. Homework should be done at a specific time each day.
- ◆ 2. Set up a place. The place should be a comfortable, quiet work place with no TV, good lighting, and, preferably, with a desk.
- ◆ 3. Break up assignments into steps.
- ◆ 4. Never use homework as a punishment.

A routine establishes a habit and develops responsibility. In step two, the place where the child works should be a special place where he or she will not be disturbed, perhaps in the bedroom or at the dining room table. There should be little distraction. One parent told me that she had her son working in the kitchen, but he would continually get up to make a snack or watch her make dinner.

Step three discusses that homework should be broken up into steps since many times the dyslexic child has a difficult time following long, complicated steps. Finally, homework should never be used as a punishment, since then the child will have ill feelings towards homework, making the experience less enjoyable. Parents can give verbal praise when the work is done. This can be done effectively when parents look over the work. If a large percentage of the work is done incorrectly, then take the time to sit down with your child and go over it.

When a child receives one-on-one help with a knowledgeable person, it can affect the progress of remediation.

Dyslexia Centers

Some dyslexic children may benefit from attending a center after school where they interact one-on-one with a trained specialist who engages the child in activities to specifically meet the needs of that child. Funding for these centers can be an issue, but parents should inquire about special assistance. When a child receives one-on-one help with a knowledgeable person it can affect the progress of remediation. A competent, trained person, knows exactly how to alleviate the patterns of dyslexia (Huston, 1992). At a dyslexic center, a child can accomplish a great deal in a reasonable amount of time. The specialist has the materials needed to give the child a beneficial experience. Finally, with parents working and having little time in the day, the child can get the attention that he or she needs to feel success and reward. For further information, parents, and teachers may want to contact the professional organizations listed at the end of this book on page 76.

Concluding Remarks

Parents of a child who has been diagnosed with dyslexia, need to realize that the diagnosis does not mean that their child cannot learn. It simply means that their child needs to find other strategies that will help him or her learn a little bit easier. The more the parents become involved in the child's life, the easier this situation will be. In addition, parents should reach out to organizations that can give them information and support. While the child needs support from the parents, the parents need support as well. Getting involved with other parents of dyslexic children can reduce the amount of anxiety and stress (Hartwig, 1984). Finally, parents should remember that the child with dyslexia can be very bright and may have many gifts which should be given an opportunity to shine. While there may be emotions of frustration and failure, the child and the parent must be persistent and continue to strive for success.

Role of the Teacher

Helping the Dyslexic Child

There are five learning principles which the teacher can keep in mind to help the dyslexic child in the classroom. First, the teacher should attempt to provide methods of multiple sensory intake since the dyslexic child learns best through the integrated, simultaneous use of all the senses: eyes, ears, speech, fingers, and muscles (Orton, 1937). Second, the teacher can promote a positive outlook on reading since most dyslexic students' frustration with reading leads to a negative, poorly motivated desire to learn to read. Third, the teacher should attempt to minimize the "labeling" effect of being called dyslexic, which may damage the child's self-esteem, lowering self-expectations as well as teacher expectations. Fourth, teachers and students should allow the dyslexic child to model their correct reading patterns, working to compensate and eliminate the dyslexic reading patterns. Fifth, teachers need to reinforce fundamental reading skills, such as sound, letter, and word recognition. This is the core of the dyslexic child's problem. Dyslexic children have delays and difficulty in learning the ways in which printed symbols stand for speech and its sounds (Orton, 1937). Using these principles, the

There are five learning principles which the teacher can keep in mind to help the dyslexic child in the classroom.

teacher can create an environment, as well as apply practical approaches, that will meet the needs of the dyslexic student.

Teacher as a Coach

The classroom teacher should be seen as a coach and facilitator. The role of the teacher as a coach is to guide the child in learning to discover self-understanding as well as the meaning behind each exercise while maintaining a challenging and supportive environment. Especially when coaching the dyslexic reader, the teacher works on how to perform an unfamiliar or challenging language task (Maria, 1987). The astute teacher who coaches will develop and offer the child optional strategies to promote the child's success, rather than blame the child because he or she failed at the teacher's chosen learning strategy.

When faced with a dyslexic student in the classroom, many instructors instinctively focus on the cause of the student's reading difficulty. Many people see the term "dyslexia" as a disease implying that the child is unintelligent and unable to learn. On the contrary, a child with dyslexic reading patterns can have normal and sometimes high intelligence. The child is capable of learning, although conventional strategies may not work. Orton and Hinshelwood, as previously mentioned, both recognize that even though it is possible that dyslexia is neurologically based, the treatment must be educational (Richardson, 1989).

An important aspect of coaching is knowing the students personally. Background information from each student is helpful in guiding each student's learning. This information can be obtained through questionnaires with older children and interviews with younger children. Questions teachers can ask are:

- ◆ What are your favorite hobbies?
- ◆ Does anyone help you with your homework?
- ◆ What is your best academic strength?
- ◆ What is your most difficult area of learning?
- ◆ What special qualities do you have?
- ◆ What do you do when faced with a difficult task?
- ◆ Is there something you could teach the class to do?

Teachers should evaluate each child's individual qualities and abilities while also being aware of each child's needs. When a teacher becomes aware of students' abilities and strengths that contribute to the learning environment, then instructional lessons can be designed specifically for the given population. Educators as coaches should adopt attitudes that teaching is a continuous experiment and open their eyes to what the children are doing, can do, and might be sensitively guided to achieve (Tierney, Readence, & Dishner, 1990).

Setting Student Goals

When the students begin to sense that they are in a nonjudgmental environment, they start to trust the teacher as a real coach who helps them achieve their goals (Moffett and Wagner, 1992). Developing personal goals helps motivate the learner. The goal system allows the teacher to defer responsibility for the child's learning to the child. For the dyslexic child goal setting is very important since it teaches responsibility and keeps the teacher informed of the child's progress. New goals can be made every quarter or semester. For example, on a quarter system the teacher may choose to have the children set or renew three goals each quarter:

◆ Personal Goal ◆ Academic Goal ◆ Home Goal

In listing each goal, the child should discuss how the goals will be met. The personal goal might be to avoid fights, have confidence in what one does, or play better on the volleyball team. The academic goals should be specific and realistic such as turn in homework on time, or use capital letters in writing. Home goals can focus on responsibility, such as cleaning one's room every other day, or focus on personal relationships, such as not talking back to mom. The personal and home goals are important since teachers need to be aware of all the areas of the dyslexic student's life. Charts can be made that keep track of how the goals are being kept. Finally, rewards can be given to those who consistently accomplish their goals. The goal system is one method of guiding the students to become aware of their own learning processes, with the student taking over more of the responsibility of learning.

Developing a Student-Centered Environment

Teachers should also see themselves in the role of developing a student-centered environment. The dyslexic child experiences more success in a student-centered environment because the structure of the lessons allows each child to actively participate, while the attitude of the teacher promotes a student's self-initiative and confidence. It is generally accepted that the student-centered environment is beneficial for students of all abilities.

> For the dyslexic child goal setting is very important since it teaches responsibility and keeps the teacher informed of the child's progress.

This example shows how adjusting instruction can sometimes help a frustrated child understand and accomplish the task. A teacher who has the needs of the students in mind tailors the instruction to fit these needs (Meyerson & Van Vactor, 1992). When a teacher observes a dyslexic child failing at a writing activity, the teacher should first try to re-explain the activity. If the child continues to fail, the teacher should try alternative methods of instructing, such as copying down the assignment for the child or demonstrating the activity so the child may model the teacher. Many children with dyslexic patterns need to have the activity broken down in steps. To merely recognize the failure with the activity, rather than try a new angle of explanation, effectively excuses the dyslexic child from performing. Without a teacher thinking in student-centered terms, the student may see him or herself as incapable of performing the task. In order to have effective programs, the classroom should be a place where activities are played out, evaluated, and adjusted.

> To merely recognize the failure with the activity, rather than try a new angle of explanation, effectively excuses the dyslexic child from performing.

Another example shows how a teacher can encourage the dyslexic child to participate in learning. During a reading activity, the student may have difficulty with vocabulary. The student asks the teacher what the word means and the teacher shows the student how to look up the word in the dictionary. Next time the student comes across an unfamiliar word, the teacher asks, "How could you find out what that word means?" The teacher watches the student look up the word, giving assistance if needed, and praises the student for his or her success. The example may appear simple, yet a remarkable number of teachers prefer to tell the dyslexic student what the word means, circumventing the student's opportunity for self-initiative.

Concluding Remarks

Coaching, counseling, and consulting are roles teachers have always wanted and they are what make education work. With the new teacher role, the more "self-directing" the students become, the freer the teacher is to counsel and coach the students toward higher levels of language learning (Moffett & Wagner, 1992). When dyslexic students are present, the teacher needs to focus attention on how each child in the classroom performs under varying conditions and tailor conditions so they are most likely to facilitate learning. Although it may be easier to set up or orchestrate an authoritative, teacher-centered environment, it does not accommodate specific learning differences. By definition, the classroom is for the students and should be centered around their needs. The teacher as a coach seeks to create a classroom as a team, with each member necessary and important, where the community is stronger than the individual, yet each individual is unique and special.

Reinforcing
Fundamental Skills

Whole Language or Phonics?

The following chapter is designed to help the teacher reinforce fundamental reading skills for dyslexic students. An ongoing debate in education concerns whether to use a phonics or whole-language approach to teach reading. While the phonics bottom-up approach focuses on learning reading skills through a basal program, the whole-language top-down approach focuses on making meaning through the use of children's literature. The teacher with the dyslexic student should combine the insights of research on whole language with the insights from skills instruction and develop an interactive model mixing both (Heymsfeld, 1992). Through the use of literature, a child will have potential for developing higher reader motivation. With instruction on word analysis skills, the child will be able to compensate for or eliminate dyslexic reading patterns and become a better reader.

Children should learn to read through a whole-language approach, but the dyslexic child may not fit into this population because dyslexic reading patterns interfere with the meaning-making

> Through the use of literature, a child will have potential for developing higher reader motivation.

29

process. While a dyslexic child is reading, he or she cannot simply skip unknown words and read on to gain meaning because too many words might be skipped. In addition, the child is not learning how to eliminate letter and word reversals and omissions. On the contrary, too often we see teachers only use mundane, skill-based activities which the dyslexic child may perceive as uninteresting and meaningless. While reading skills are being developed, they should be taught in the context of meaningful text through the literature read in the class. Therefore, the emphasis should not be on simply teaching phonics or whole language, but on teaching the word analysis skills in a meaning based context.

Word Analysis

Word analysis is the skill of analyzing the word, knowing it is pronunciation, spelling, and meaning. The purpose of learning methods of word analysis is to assist the students in developing automatic use of these skills. Once these skills are learned, students can transform the text for meaning. The teacher with the dyslexic student needs to teach these skills so the dyslexic student can compensate for dyslexic reading patterns with the ultimate goal of eliminating them. Once the dyslexic child learns these skills, the goal is to free his or her mental energy to focus on the primary purpose of reading, constructing meaning and developing personal interpretation (Ruddell, in press; Commeyras, 1993; Heymsfeld, 1992; Genishi, 1988; Maria, 1987).

When skills are taught in a meaningful context, the dyslexic student is more likely to remember them.

Word analysis skills should be taught in a meaningful context. This is important since dyslexic students have difficulty retaining information. When skills are taught in a meaningful context, the dyslexic student is more likely to remember them. Four skills used in the analysis of words will be discussed that are especially vital for a dyslexic child: letter recognition, phonemic awareness, letter patterns, and use of context clues. What follows is a further description of the skills and suggested activities used to build these skills.

Letter Recognition

Letter recognition is a word analysis skill which identifies and recognizes the letters in the alphabet. The purpose of letter recognition is to be able to learn how to read, write, and communicate with language. Using strategies to teach these skills is extremely helpful for the teacher with a dyslexic student since this student is many times delayed in learning letter recognition. In addition, dyslexic reading patterns, such as reversals, make learning letter identification more difficult.

Before instruction takes place, the teacher should first find out what the dyslexic student already knows. Marie Clay (1979) discusses several ways of doing this with a letter identification survey. A letter identification survey is when a teacher shows a child the alphabet, scrambled up, points to a letter, and asks the student what the letter is. The letters are scrambled up to discern the student's true recognition, because many children learn the alphabet song long before they enter school and can repeat the letters in order, regardless of whether they recognize them. Letters should be written in uppercase and lowercase.

If the student lacks total letter identification, the teacher can begin teaching the letter names with alphabet books, songs, and chants (Ruddell, in press). Alphabet books should be colorful and interesting. Older students can be encouraged to make alphabet books for the younger students to read and take home with them. Rhymes and songs are highly motivating and a great way for dyslexic students to learn letters because they are multisensory and easy to retain.

Phonemic Awareness

Phonemic awareness is the word analysis skill of being able to use letter-sound correspondence to read and spell words. A phoneme is the smallest sound unit in language. Dyslexic students need to be able to direct and focus attention on the separate sounds in a given word so that they will eventually be able to read fluently (Ruddell, in press). Teachers with dyslexic students need to use strategies when teaching phonemic awareness since these students may have difficulty with auditory distinction.

An activity known as Elkonin boxes (from Russian D.B. Elkonis) can be used by a teacher with a dyslexic child who appears to have difficulty with phonemic awareness. The goal of the activity is to help the student think about the order of sounds in spoken simple words using multisensory intake. After a story is read in class, the teacher can use the following steps with words from the story.

- ◆ 1. Provide the child with a picture of a familiar, simple object such as a cat, ship, or bus that was read about in the story.
- ◆ 2. Pronounce the word slowly for the child, deliberately articulating the word. The child should watch the teacher's lips as the word is said.
- ◆ 3. Ask the child to pronounce the word aloud. Ask the child to say the word slowly.

> Rhymes and songs are highly motivating and a great way for dyslexic students to learn letters because they are multisensory and easy to retain.

◆ 4. Have a sectioned card that has the exact number of squares as the word has sounds. For example, the word cat has three sounds, c-a-t, so this should be done with a card with three squares. Articulate the word slowly and place a counter or button into each square of the sectioned card sound by sound.

◆ 5. Ask the child to repeat the word slowly, pronounce it, and place a counter in each square as a sound is said. If the task is too difficult for the child, the teacher can model it again or place a finger on the child's finger and help him or her through the task. In addition, the teacher can have the child articulate the word as the teacher places the counters. All approximations should be accepted.

◆ 6. Ask the child to read the sentence where the word was found in the story and practice the same procedure.

◆ 7. Select another word from the same story, provide another picture, and follow the same modeling procedure.

Rhyming books use repetitious patterns that make reading enjoyable and easier.

Gradually, the responsibility should be transferred over to the student so that it becomes automatic. A student can be more challenged with this activity by covering a word so that only the first phoneme is showing. Griffith and Olson (1992) suggest that the words for this activity be chosen from text that the dyslexic student is reading. This is helpful since the student is learning words in the context of reading.

Letter Pattern Recognition

Letter patterns are syllables in multisyllabic words such as "at" in "bat" or "ous" in "house." Graphemes, or letter patterns, are organized into consonants or vowel patterns. The reason letter patterns are taught is to increase rapid word analysis (Ruddell, in press). Teachers with dyslexic students should reinforce the child's letter pattern recognition since these students have difficulty identifying and recalling letter sounds. A strategy teachers can use is rhyme.

Rhyming books use repetitious patterns that make reading enjoyable and easier. Rhyming is the most natural way to learn to group words by their sounds. Students with dyslexia can develop an awareness of the connection between sound categories and alphabetic code through practice with rhymes (Bradley, 1991). Not only is it an enjoyable way to learn, but rhyming helps students predict what is coming next. Predictable books can also be used for the purpose of letter pattern recognition. There are various books on the market that contain letter patterns and rhyme. Instruction from the text can be used to increase word analysis.

For example, when working with a dyslexic student alone or in a group, the teacher can use a *Mother Goose* story which is filled with excellent rhymes. The teacher can begin by reading the story aloud to the student. It is important to read with rhythm, almost as though it were a song, while modeling correct reading patterns. After the first reading, the teacher should ask the child if he or she noticed anything special about the ends of the sentences. If the child does not offer a response, then the teacher reads an example of two sentences that rhyme and asks the child the same question again. For example, the teacher may read "Humpty Dumpty sat on a <u>wall</u>. Humpty Dumpty had a great <u>fall</u>." The teacher explains to the child that the endings of the sentences, <u>wall</u> and <u>fall</u>, rhyme, or have the same sound pattern, "all." The teacher re-reads the book again, encouraging the child to follow along and point out the patterns. Finally, the teacher can have the child read the story. The child may simply read from memory, using the rhyme to predict what comes next, which helps develop recognition of the letter patterns.

Using Context Clues

Context clues are indicators in a story that reveal what words mean. The purpose of context clues is to aid in word identification and comprehension during reading. When working with students with dyslexia who have difficulty sounding out words, context clues can help reveal what the word is much quicker and with less frustration. In the end, the student not only reads faster but has a more positive outlook on reading.

Two activities that can be used by the teacher with the dyslexic student in small groups or with the whole class are a "cloze" or a "mask." A cloze activity allows the teacher to help dyslexic students use context to form hypotheses about unknown words (Gillet & Temple, 1990). The steps for a cloze activity are:

◆ 1. Teacher selects a book to read to the class. The book should be predictable and enjoyable.

◆ 2. The book is read aloud by the teacher or by the students several times so that the students are familiar with the book.

◆ 3. The teacher writes out the text, leaving certain words blank. These deletions can follow patterns. It can be a selective word deletion such as important nouns, verbs, adverbs, or adjectives; a systematic word deletion such as all the third, fourth, or fifth words in the text; or a partial word deletion such as deleting the whole word except for the first letter.

◆ 4. The students read through the written text and fill in words that make sense.

> When working with students with dyslexia who have difficulty sounding out words, context clues can help reveal what the word is much quicker and with less frustration.

33

The students use illustrations, the meaning of the sentence, or the surrounding words to figure out the blank words. Students should be taught how to do a cloze activity with modeling and explanation.

In the mask activity the teacher follows the same steps of a cloze activity. The only difference is that in step three, the teacher puts sticky notes over the words on the actual book. Big books can be used for a mask activity since it is easier to put sticky notes over the words. The teacher can ask how the student knew what the word was. If the student gives a different word that means the same thing, it should be accepted. Cloze and mask activities are fun for students and can be used at different reading levels.

Dealing with Unfamiliar Words

Teachers can post the following steps in the classroom to remind students of different strategies to use during reading when they get to an unfamiliar word.

◆ 1. Read the sentence in which the word is found and use the text clues, pictures, or other words in the sentence to figure out what the word is.

◆ 2. Look at letter patterns that are familiar to you and try to sound them out.

◆ 3. Break up the word into sounds or phonemes, using a finger or thumb. Try to pronounce each phoneme one at a time and re-read the sentence with the word. For example, with the word remarkable read re - mark - a - ble, covering all the sounds with a thumb except the one that is being read.

◆ 4. With larger words, look for smaller words that are familiar inside the larger word. For example, in the word intelligent there are the words in and tell.

◆ 5. Skip the word, keep reading, and try to make meaning from the text.

◆ 6. Check to see how important the word is to the meaning of the text. Ask a peer or the teacher for help.

Each step can be modeled for the dyslexic student so that the use becomes automatic. The main goal of these steps is for the dyslexic student to try out various methods first, before relying on someone else to simply tell him or her what the word is. These strategies help develop an understanding of language and how it works. Again, a teacher should not force the strategy on the child but rather introduce the strategy and then let the child explore what works for him or her.

If the student gives a different word that means the same thing, it should be accepted.

Metacognition

Metacognition is self-regulation of some form of thinking and learning activity. In reading, metacognition is knowledge that each person is in charge of his or her learning. This involves self-knowledge and self-monitoring of comprehension and progress (Vacca, Vacca, & Gove, 1991). The goal of metacognition is for the student to have increased awareness of his or her reading process. The child sees what strategies work and why and gains a better understanding of the material.

Teachers with dyslexic students in the classroom can promote metacognition by using multisensory intake and modeling successful strategies. One way this is done is by activating background knowledge. Activating background knowledge is when the teacher brings the student's previous experiences into focus first before starting any reading at all. By doing this, the teacher is giving the student a ground floor to work from. Knowledge is activated and other learning will follow. By the time a student enters first grade, a great deal of knowledge has already developed. To disregard all this knowledge and experience would detract from a student's learning experience. Therefore, teachers need to learn to activate students' prior knowledge in order to assist students in the meaning construction process (Ruddell, in press; Vacca, Vacca, & Gove, 1991; Routman, 1988; Maria, 1987).

> In reading, metacognition is knowledge that each person is in charge of his or her learning.

SAIL Program

The SAIL (Students Achieving Independent Learning) Program, started by Janet L. Bergman (1992), is a metacognitive program which has students set goals for learning, learn reading strategies, use the strategies while reading, and then evaluate how well the strategies work. The focus of the program is for low-achieving readers to successfully and independently read. SAIL is a program to promote frequent and extensive student reading, increase student motivation, and improve reading ability (Bergman, 1992). For the teacher with dyslexic students, the SAIL program helps by promoting a positive outlook on reading, modeling correct reading strategies, and shifting responsibility over to the student. The more the student interacts with the text, the more he or she will realize ways to make the process occur more fluently.

First, the teacher has the students devise their own personal goals for improving their reading abilities. This can be specific or general, depending on what areas the student has difficulty with: word omission, word reversals, or word analysis.

Second, the teacher teaches strategies that help the students monitor understanding and solve problems during reading by visualizing, thinking aloud, summarizing, and making predictions. This begins with extensive modeling and coaching support from the teacher. The teacher's assistance diminishes over time as the students become more competent and independent readers, thinkers, and learners.

Third, while the child is reading, he or she selects a strategy to use. After reading, the student then verifies what strategy was used and why. The list below of questions to ask during reading can be displayed in the class so that when children read, they can refer to the list to help activate strategy use (Bergman, 1992). These questions focus on metacognition. In order to accommodate the students' languages, some students may want to word the strategies differently or add new ones. The important thing is to observe and make note of what works well for the child, so that he or she reads with less frustration and more enthusiasm.

> The teacher's assistance diminishes over time as the students become more competent and independent readers, thinkers, and learners.

Below is a sample of Bergman's (1992) SAIL reading strategies, listed in the form of questions, that can be posted in the classroom:

◆ 1. *To get the gist of the story:* What is the story about? What is the problem? What is the solution? What makes me think so?

◆ 2. *To predict, verify, and decide:* What's going to happen next? Is my prediction still good? Do I need to change my prediction? What makes me think so?

◆ 3. *To visualize, verify, and decide:* What does this (person, place, thing) look like? Is the picture in my mind still good? Do I need to change my picture? What makes me think so?

◆ 4. *To summarize the story:* What's happened so far? What makes me think so?

◆ 5. *To think aloud about the story:* What am I thinking? Why?

◆ 6. *To solve problems when I don't understand:* Shall I guess? Ignore and read on? Re-read or look back? Why should I use that strategy?

The list is clear and easy to understand so that the students can monitor their own reading process by asking themselves these questions while they read.

The goal of SAIL is for the child to become a motivated, independent and self-regulated learner (Gaskins, 1992). If the program is done with partners, useful interaction takes place among the students while they interpret the text. Again, this gives the dyslexic student a chance to correct reading patterns, while providing another sensory medium (oral communication) for conveying the meaning of the words and story. In an environment where active comprehension is promoted, students will learn to discuss with one another what the story is about and why they think so. During the discussions, students can be put in small groups in order to talk in detail about the story. While the SAIL program explicitly teaches reading and thinking strategies, the child decides what learning approach to use. Learning to use strategies is a meaningful task for students because it helps them become better readers (Bergman, 1992).

PLEASE Program

One of the most frustrating hurdles for the dyslexic child is the acquisition of writing skills since dyslexic reading patterns can affect writing as well. The dyslexic child usually finds the complex demands of writing burdensome.

Marshall Welch (1992) devised a process-oriented approach that specifically helps the needs of children with mild learning disabilities. While there is research that suggests the writing process should be shaped by the student (Graves, 1983), the dyslexic child often experiences overwhelming frustration and anxiety when confronted with language arts activities. Since dyslexia affects how a child identifies, pronounces, and uses different speech sounds in language, the difficulty will also take place when the dyslexic child tries to write down these sounds. While Welch's suggestions are by no means the only way to facilitate writing, they can begin the writing process for dyslexic students by easing their anxiety.

The goal of the program is to help students learn to monitor and orchestrate the cognitive activities involved in the process of writing.

The goal of the program is to help students learn to monitor and orchestrate the cognitive activities involved in the process of writing. The process establishes strategies that facilitate metacognitive problem solving and provide students with a repertoire of behaviors through the use of a first letter mnemonic that cues the students on how to complete the writing task independently.

The program consists of six steps that are explicitly taught to the students before any of the writing begins:

P = Pick a topic.
L = List your ideas about the topic.
E = Evaluate your list.
A = Activate paragraph with a topic sentence.
S = Supply supporting sentences.
E = End with a concluding sentence.

While not all paragraphs have to begin with a topic sentence, some students have difficulty organizing their thoughts and, therefore, a structured approach can be an effective way to start. Once the students are more comfortable with writing, they can practice different ways of beginning paragraphs. The steps are simple, clear, and easy for the dyslexic child to handle. In addition, the dyslexic child will have an easier time with the task if it is broken down into steps.

The instructor should begin by modeling the process for the students and then have them practice with a partner to create an essay. The essays can be shared in small groups that discuss the process, what worked, and why. Too often it is assumed that writing will come naturally to all students. The dyslexic child who experiences frustration in elementary school may have these feelings throughout high school and college. The PLEASE program relieves some of that frustration by laying out specific guidelines that assist the student with pre-writing, planning, composing, and revising essays. While these are only suggestions and do not have to be used in all writing, the steps are useful in helping a dyslexic student produce a comprehensive piece of work.

Concluding Remarks

While the whole-language approach is advocated by many educators, the child with dyslexia is not necessarily able to use whole-language approaches to learn how to read and write. The dyslexic child is dealing with learning patterns that need to be addressed. The sensitive teacher must realize that the dyslexic child will have a more successful experience if skills instruction is reinforced in a meaningful context. With the use of literature and the activities suggested, teachers can teach the dyslexic child how to identify, pronounce, and use different speech sounds and written symbols in language.

> The instructor should begin by modeling the process for the students and then have them practice with a partner to create an essay.

Classroom Methods for Teaching Language Arts

Effective Techniques

The following chapter will discuss four techniques for teaching language arts with a dyslexic student in the classroom: Shared Reading, Guided Reading, Peer Teaching, and Cross-Age Tutoring. The four activities can be used for general classroom teaching, while also promoting principles that allow the child with dyslexic reading patterns to participate and feel successful.

Shared Reading

Shared reading is most useful for younger students, grades kindergarten through third, because the text is read repeatedly. The teacher activates background knowledge on a topic, reads a book on that topic, and then asks the students comprehension questions about the book. The goals are for the child to develop a positive impression of reading and eventually read the text independently. The steps of the shared reading process help the teacher with a dyslexic student in the classroom by promoting a positive outlook on reading and modeling correct reading patterns. Our basic concept of classroom reading is having thirty children reading silently at their desks. This

> The goals are for the child to develop a positive impression of reading and eventually read the text independently.

can be intensely frustrating for the dyslexic child. Shared reading is a high energy, enjoyable time where the students interact with one another and the text in a nonthreatening environment (Routman, 1988).

Shared reading is especially helpful for a dyslexic child in the classroom. Because of prior failure, dyslexic children are often uninterested in reading, finding it a burdensome chore. Shared reading helps the child to experience the fulfillment of understanding a story's meaning. The activity provides a high level of support from the instructor and teaches the child that what he or she can do with help, he or she can eventually do alone (Depree & Iversen, 1993). This is supported by Vygotsky (1962) who developed the term "scaffolding." Scaffolding is the idea that the more practiced student is to assist the learner until the learner reaches competency. The dyslexic student works in partnership with the classmate who scaffolds the task by engaging in appropriate instructional interactions. As the dyslexic student increases in competency and control over the task, the responsibility moves more to that student.

Scaffolding is the idea that the more practiced student is to assist the learner until the learner reaches competency.

The steps of a shared reading activity can be altered according to the purpose of the activity and the needs of the students. As a framework the teacher initially takes on the responsibility of reading and gradually hands it over to the students. The following shared reading activity promotes active participation with the use of exciting literature.

- ◆ STEP 1: Select the text
- ◆ STEP 2: Activate background knowledge
- ◆ STEP 3: Read text aloud
- ◆ STEP 4: Solicit students' initial responses
- ◆ STEP 5: Second reading by the teacher with discussion
- ◆ STEP 6: Third reading with individual copies

In step 1, the teacher selects the text to use. Shared reading gives the teacher the opportunity to use more difficult reading material with his or her students since the teacher is doing the reading. Johnson and Louis (1990) advocate material that is meaningful, memorable, repetitive, rhythmic, structured, energetic, and of good literary quality. When the material is repetitive and rhythmic, classroom students, including the dyslexic child, are more likely to remember the text and more likely to remember the meaning of each word. Predictable books, which are books where students can guess what happens next, are also very effective since the children can begin to see patterns in language and learn through repetition.

In step 2, the teacher activates students' background knowledge on the book's topic. The most common method is to brainstorm the idea or topic. (Depree & Iversen, 1993; Routman, 1988; Ruddell, in press; Maria, 1987). On the following page there is an example of how to ask the students questions that touch on certain themes of the book before the text is read. The questions open up the children's own personal experiences and activate background knowledge. Another way to introduce the text is to show the cover of the book and ask the students for predictions about the story (Depree & Iversen, 1993).

In step 3, the teacher reads the book aloud to the students, promoting a positive outlook on reading and modeling correct reading patterns. The teacher has the only copy of the book. The idea is not to have the children focus on the letters and words, but merely to listen to the story. The activity should provide a setting similar to a parent reading aloud to his or her children (Holdaway, 1982). The teacher should read the story with inflection and enthusiasm, emphasizing the plot and meaning of the text. Essentially, the teacher gives the message of the book to the children without the children having to decipher that message by reading the words. Because the meaning is conveyed without reading letters and words, the dyslexic child is as involved in the story as the other students.

The teacher should read the story with inflection and enthusiasm, emphasizing the plot and meaning of the text.

In step 4, the students respond to the story. The teacher should ask questions which ensure that the child has paid attention and understands the story. The questions are generally basic: "What did you like best about the story?" "Who are the main characters in the book?" "What is illustrated in this picture?" "What did the main character do?"

In step 5, the teacher reads the story a second time. During this reading the teacher works on teaching and reinforcing fundamental reading skills, such as the direction in which the words are read, sounds in words, and strategies for figuring out new words. During the second reading of the story, it is often useful for the teacher to read out of a "big book" encouraging students to follow along (Depree & Iversen, 1993). During this second reading it is not only important to check for understanding but also to promote higher levels of thinking through the use of interpretive, applicative, and transactive questioning. For example, teachers can ask students to answer why a character did an action or answer whether they would have done the same thing.

The Cowardly and the Brave

Answer questions 1, 2, 3, and 4 before you read *Cowardly Clyde*. Complete the rest of the questionnaire after you have finished the story.

The Brave

1. Define what it means to be brave. _____
_____
_____

2. Give an example of something a brave person would do. _____
_____
_____

3. How do you think the world views people who are brave? _____
_____
_____

4. Would you consider yourself to be brave? _____
   Give at least one good example to support your opinion.
_____
_____

NOW READ *Cowardly Clyde.*
5. What makes Sir Galavant brave? _____
_____
_____

6. What makes Clyde brave? _____
_____
_____

7. Is Clyde happier being cowardly or brave? Why?_____
_____

8. On the back of this page, write a dialogue between Sir Galavant and Clyde in which Sir Galavant admits that being brave is not all that it is said to be. Perform your dialogue with a partner for the class.

9. How would this story be different if Clyde was the brave one and Sir Galavant cowardly? Write one page from this "new" story.

Reprinted from TCM354 Literature Activities for Reluctant Readers, *Teacher Created Materials, 1991*

In step 6, the final reading takes place with each student having his or her own copy of the story. This time students read the text on their own. After the entire activity, make the books available during free reading time.

Shared reading opens up the reading experience to all students in a nonthreatening environment with challenging text and with the teacher encouraging risk taking. The dyslexic child can follow along and not only hear the text, but begin to make the connection between speech and print. The exercise benefits the teacher with a dyslexic child in the classroom because in addition to teaching all students, the dyslexic child is guided by being able to model the teacher's correct reading patterns.

Guided Silent Reading

Guided silent reading is most useful for students in grades four and up since the students must be able to read silently. The teacher activates background knowledge on the topic of a book, has students make predictions about that book, has students silently read sections from the book, and then asks comprehension questions about the section read. The goal in a guided silent reading activity is to promote independent reading and the ability to assess the content of the story.

The goal in a guided silent reading activity is to promote independent reading and the ability to assess the content of the story.

Guided reading activities have been used in the classroom for many years and are also sometimes called Directed Reading Activities (DRA). The difference in this approach is that it is structured in a way to particularly help the dyslexic student silently read interesting material, actively comprehend what is being read, and comprehend the meaning of the story.

Six suggested steps for a guided silent reading activity in the classroom are listed below and then described in detail.

◆ STEP 1: Choose the text.
◆ STEP 2: Choose the idea to brainstorm.
◆ STEP 3: Show the cover and make predictions.
◆ STEP 4: Think about the idea.
◆ STEP 5: Read the text.
◆ STEP 6: Check for comprehension.

In step one, the teacher chooses a text that is at the average student's instructional level, meaning the student reads the text with 90% accuracy. If a book is too difficult for the dyslexic student, he or she will not be able to keep up. Books should also be interesting so that students are motivated to read about the topic. Dyslexic students will be particularly encouraged to read if the book is on a topic that they are interested in. In addition, the book should be predictable. When books are predictable, the students finish a section and want to read on to verify what they believe will happen next.

In step two, the teacher brainstorms an idea that is crucial to the book by evoking student discussion on the topic. Again, apply the idea to a student's personal experiences in order to activate the child's background knowledge (Vacca, Vacca, & Gove, 1991). When background information is activated, then the student already understands the story's meaning before the reading process even begins (Routman, 1988). All comments on the idea should be accepted and written down on a poster or the chalkboard.

In step three, the teacher shows the cover of the book. Since many students are visual learners, the cover can activate more ideas. For the dyslexic child, the cover picture is an alternative sensory intake mechanism which will help generate prereading ideas and expectations of the story. The teacher should solicit predictions about the story, where it takes place, who it is about and what might happen. The teacher should also ask for comments about the title: "What does the title tell you about the story?"

In step four, the teacher gives the students an idea to think about before they begin reading. For the dyslexic student this step not only gives more focus to the content of the story but also motivation to want to read on (Depree & Iversen, 1993). For example, when reading *Island of the Blue Dolphins* by Scott O'Dell (1960), the idea in step three might be "survival" while the idea for the reading of the first chapter might be "life on an island."

In step five, the students read the text silently. Depending on the length of the story, the teacher may have a student read all of the text or sections. Silent reading allows a dyslexic student to begin reading independently and feel more comfortable with reading since no one else will be listening. During the silent reading, the teacher should be observing the strategies the students use while they read, especially the dyslexic child. For example, is the student tracking and following the text with his or her finger? Does the student sound out difficult words, ask for help with an unfamiliar word, or continually look off into space and turn pages? If the child is distracted, then the teacher should approach the child and try to get him or her back on track. When students read at different paces, simple activities can be available for the students who finish first. For example, have a thought or question on the board for the students to answer about the story, have the students read the section twice, or have them draw a picture of what they read.

In step six, the teacher needs to check for comprehension. This is especially important with the dyslexic students since the teacher needs to make sure the student actually read the section and understood what it was about. Questions can be asked orally with the whole class, students can discuss the questions in groups, or they can write down the answers independently. It is best when all approaches are used periodically throughout the story. More importantly, the teacher needs to vary the type of questions asked. Types of questions include:

◆ *Factual*: ask specific facts about the story such as who, what, where, when, and how.

◆ *Interpretive:* ask for an explanation about why things happened the way they did in the story. Ask students to read between the lines.

◆ *Analytical:* ask students to analyze what they read, to think about the story's significance, and to tell what the story means to them.

◆ *Transactive:* ask students to take on the role of a character and discuss what they would have done in that character's shoes in a certain situation.

◆ *Predictive:* ask student to guess what will happen next in the story.

As a comprehension check the students can be asked to retell what they have read. This also helps the dyslexic student with sequencing events.

Many dyslexic students are not given the opportunity to actively engage in literature since some educators are worried that they may be incapable of doing the activity. However, all students have the capability to actively engage in the text, and when doing so with pre-reading activities and follow-up activities, the process takes on very significant meaning for that student. The shared reading activity allows the dyslexic students to observe how other students' reading strategies are used. It allows them to model these correct reading patterns. Overall, this is very useful in the learning process, since the guided silent reading activity allows the student to take on even more responsibility.

Peer Teaching

Peer teaching is when one student in the classroom helps another student. The goal of peer teaching is to have a high achieving student help the low achieving student. This is particularly helpful for the teacher in the classroom with a dyslexic student since the teacher cannot attend to the needs of the dyslexic student as readily as possible. When students can share solutions and help each other in the classroom, dyslexic students can enjoy the learning experience with less frustration and anxiety. This promotes a more positive outlook on reading. In addition, the dyslexic student has the opportunity to model the peer's correct reading patterns.

The best way to promote peer teaching with the dyslexic student in the classroom is to seat the student with dyslexic reading patterns next to a high achieving student who has a friendly outlook on learning. Some students may be high achievers in the classroom yet unlikely to share solutions and successful strategies with others. In addition, it is important to avoid seating the dyslexic student next to someone who may tease him or her about his or her difficulties.

There are many benefits from peer teaching for the dyslexic student. First, when a teacher has more than thirty students in the class, it is difficult to meet the individual needs of all the students all the time. Students with dyslexia can be more demanding than other students, and their needs should be met in order to avoid frustration, failure, and lack of motivation. Ideally, when the teacher knows that a knowledgeable, more capable student is in the next seat, the teacher is assured that the dyslexic student is given help when he or she needs it.

Second, students with dyslexic reading patterns might feel more comfortable asking a peer for help instead of raising their hands in class. Dyslexic students usually do not want others to know about their difficulty. Many times students simply do not ask for help because they do not want anyone to know they do not understand. With peer teaching, the label of being a student who always needs extra help is minimized. When a dyslexic student is sitting next to someone who can answer a question, he or she will be more inclined to ask for help.

Third, when the dyslexic student sits next to a high achieving peer, he or she models correct reading patterns and successful learning strategies. Some students learn simply by watching the proper method. In this situation, less attention is drawn to the fact that the dyslexic student may not know how to do the activity.

> **When a dyslexic student is sitting next to someone who can answer a question, he or she will be more inclined to ask for help.**

An example of peer teaching can be seen with a reading comprehension activity. All the students in the class are asked to read a
poem silently to themselves. During reading, if the dyslexic student
is unfamiliar with a word, he or she can ask the peer sitting in the
next seat the word's definition or pronunciation. This eliminates the
fear of raising a hand in class when everyone else is reading.

The teacher can talk to the peer beforehand and train him or her on
how to interact with the dyslexic student. The peer will feel a sense
of importance in working as a teacher. Finally, the students are
asked to write a paragraph on what they liked and did not like about
the poem. The dyslexic student and peer can discuss their ideas
together.

Teachers need to realize that most dyslexic students might not want
to participate in an activity. But with peer teaching, they are
involved and learning. In addition, the student is receiving one-on-
one help which is difficult for the busy teacher to give. One important factor with peer teaching is that the teacher must carefully select
the peer and discuss with the peer and the dyslexic student the structure of the relationship.

> Cross-age tutoring is
> when a child from an
> upper grade works
> with a child in a lower
> grade on an activity
> during school time.

Cross-Age Tutoring

Cross-age tutoring is when a child from an upper grade works with
a child in a lower grade on an activity during school time. The goal
is for the older student to reinforce fundamental reading skills and
promote a positive outlook on reading while the younger student
receives one-on-one attention. Cross-age tutoring will help the
teacher with the older dyslexic student in the classroom by teaching
responsibility, reinforcing fundamental reading skills, and developing positive self-esteem. Cross-age tutoring helps the teacher with
the younger dyslexic student by promoting a positive outlook on
reading, learning fundamental reading skills, and giving the student
one-on-one help.

One option available to the teacher is an ongoing program with
another class. For example, a sixth grade class might work with
kindergarten students once a week. The steps in a sample cross-age
tutoring program are:

◆ STEP 1: Coordinate with another teacher and decide which
students will participate. Teachers can choose specific
dyslexic students or have the whole class participate. Decide
when and where the students will meet. Students should
work in a place with little distractions for as long as the
young student can stay on task. Pair the students.

◆ STEP 2: Have the older students trained to be tutors with the teacher modeling. Students need to learn how to read books aloud to younger students, point out pictures during reading, and ask questions about the story.

◆ STEP 3: Have the pairs meet first and play games to break the ice so that a friendly, trusting relationship is established. It is important to pair a younger dyslexic child with a mature, older child who is patient and will not tease. With the goal of minimizing negative labeling effects in mind, the teacher may also consider whether it is even necessary to tell the older child that the younger has dyslexia.

◆ STEP 4: Have the older student select a story and practice reading before he or she meets with the younger student. The older student reads the story aloud to the younger student. As time goes by, the younger student can select the book and practice reading to the older student.

◆ STEP 5: The tutor should then have a follow-up activity about the story that might include drawing, writing, or both.

> It is important to pair a younger dyslexic child with a mature, older child who is patient and will not tease.

Cross-age tutoring is a promising way to help older and younger dyslexic readers improve their reading fluency and comprehension. The benefit gained by the older dyslexic students is that they strengthen their basic skills and improve their self-esteem (Cameron, Depree, & Walker, 1992). For dyslexic students their confidence builds, and they begin to take risks and venture forth to their fullest potential while the fear of reading slowly goes away (Gaskins, 1992). The role of the older student is that of a mentor and coach who is sensitive to frustration with reading. If the dyslexic child is the younger student, he or she gets one-on-one help and attention. While looking up to the older peer, the dyslexic student realizes that someone is supporting him or her.

Labbo and Teale (1990) conducted a study on cross-age tutoring with low-achieving fifth graders and kindergarten students. The fifth graders were trained to be tutors. They were taught how to select appropriate books, introduce the books, and discuss them with the younger students. Collaborative groups were formed with the fifth graders in order to reflect on the quality of interaction and develop strategies to improve subsequent readings. The fifth graders showed a change in their attitudes towards reading and made significant gains in their own achievement.

I had the opportunity to develop a cross-age reading program between my sixth grade and the kindergarten class at my school site. Special training and preparation took place in order to teach the sixth graders how to read to the younger children, how to ask questions, and how to be positive role models. The training is important and should be reinforced throughout the program. Certain skills were taught such as:

◆ Holding the book halfway between the child and reader.

◆ Pointing out objects the child may know.

◆ Building vocabulary.

◆ Asking the child to predict what might happen next.

The buddy program became so successful that we used buddies to walk kindergartners to assemblies, participate in physical education, do arts and crafts, cook, and teach board games. All activities included reading, writing, speaking, or listening. The sixth graders learned how to be role models and felt good about themselves. The kindergartners had big brothers or sisters to look up to and felt motivated to learn. One of the best buddy situations in the program was between a sixth grade learning-disabled student who read at a fourth grade level and a kindergartner who spoke little English. The learning-disabled student was sensitive to the boy's frustration with reading. The sixth grader was able to reinforce his own skills during the tutoring process while also developing a positive outlook on reading. He looked forward to his weekly hour when he would read to his kindergarten buddy. Both benefited greatly from the program and developed a positive relationship with each other.

> The sixth grader was able to reinforce his own skills during the tutoring process while also developing a positive outlook on reading.

Concluding Remarks

The days of sitting a child, isolated with a basal reader, are over. Rich, colorful literature motivates students to read and is readily available in bookstores and libraries. Teachers can fill the classroom with books on all topics for all reading levels so all students can find an area of interest and level of fluency. In addition, children enjoy the learning process when interacting with students in the classroom, or in other classes. The four techniques discussed in this chapter are good, basic, sound teaching methods from which all students benefit. The nondyslexic is by no means short changed in the process. It just so happens that the dyslexic particularly flourishes in this environment. Shared reading and guided reading are practical methods that can be used in the classroom to teach reading. With these methods that dyslexic student experiences less frustration because of the activation of background knowledge prior to engaging in the text. Peer teaching is a practical way for the dyslexic child to get the assistance he or she may need when the teacher is not available for one–on–one teaching. Finally, cross–age tutoring is an excellent way for two teachers at the same school to have students interact across the grade levels and help one another enjoy the learning process. All methods should be adjusted to the teacher's classroom population and teaching styles.

Classroom Methods for Teaching Content Areas

Reading Is a Gatekeeper

If the classroom has a child with dyslexia, the teacher may find that his or her inability to read does not affect achievement in other school subjects (Mayo Clinic, 1993). However, because reading is a skill basic to most other school subjects, a child with dyslexia can be at a disadvantage in other subjects. Since social studies and science involve reading and writing, the techniques used in the previous chapters can be used in these subject areas as well. Teachers need to be aware of the child's areas of need and use strategies that will help the child learn.

> Dyslexia will not affect whether a child can learn about the fifty states during social studies.

Social Studies

Dyslexia will not affect whether a child can learn about the fifty states during social studies. But, memorization and retention of that knowledge might be difficult. Therefore, a child with dyslexic patterns might need to find strategies that will help him or her with memorization. One way to deal with memorization is for the child to learn the information using all of his or her senses. For example, a child could read the names of the fifty states, write down the names of the states, listen to a jingle on the fifty states, and manipulate a puzzle of the fifty states. A child with dyslexic patterns may need to come up with tricks to use in order for the memorization to come easier, such as coming up with a mnemonic to memorize historical names and places or making up a rap when learning historical dates.

Science

Dyslexia will not affect whether a child can learn about the water cycle during science, but the sequencing of the water cycle might be difficult to learn. If this is the case, memory-enhancing methods should be used. The child can draw pictures of the water cycle or cut out pictures of the sun, rain, clouds, and river to manipulate. The child might want to read books on the water cycle or look at a short film. Again, this broadens the child's perception by providing additional methods of sensory intake. Most likely, the scientific concepts are not difficult for the dyslexic child, but rather, the concepts of memorization, sequencing, retaining information, or reading the material are. The important thing is how the information is learned.

Math

When discussing dyslexia, the subject of math is often placed in a separate category, since dyslexia is usually categorized as a reading disability. However, many children who have dyslexic patterns in their reading, also demonstrate these patterns in their math skills (Steeves, 1979). The student may understand the mathematical concept but when writing the answer reverse a number or character. Many students who are not dyslexic may exhibit these patterns. The suggestions below will help all children with mathematical difficulties, especially the dyslexic child. Other dyslexics may have strong math skills with weaknesses only in the areas of reading and writing.

Difficulty with numerals does not necessarily mean that a dyslexic student can never be a mathematician (Steeves, 1979). When working with those who have difficulty with math skill problems, many of the same language arts principles apply. The student should take an active role in the learning process and focus on the math area that is frustrating. Is the area of difficulty with writing numbers correctly, sequencing, counting, combining mathematical concepts, or a combination? The teacher should take on the role of a coach and have the learning process center around the needs of the student. A student may know that 9 x 5 = 45 but may write 54 when writing the answer. Another student may have difficulty reading the difference between a 6 and a 9. A child who may not be able to identify numbers will have difficulty in all areas of math. If the teacher is aware of the child's frustration and observes the behavior in order to identify the area of

> The student should take an active role in the learning process and focus on the math area that is frustrating.

difficulty, an instructional plan can be established that will address the child's needs. Peer teaching will be helpful. A child who is skilled in an area can help the dyslexic child with one-on-one coaching. At the same time, the skilled student is reinforcing his or her own knowledge and both students benefit.

With math, the dyslexic child should be taught using visual, kinesthetic, and auditory input (Steeves, 1979). Many dyslexic children are kinesthetic learners and cannot visualize the mathematical concepts. The best approach is to use hands-on math activities. The child who has difficulty with numbers can use block numbers with the front side colorful and the back side a dull gray. This deals with the reversal problem. The block numbers can then be arranged in sequential order. A child who has difficulty with addition can use a pile of beans and a pile of uncooked pasta and put the two together to count the total. Children will understand their multiplication tables better if, instead of saying 5 x 2 = 10, the students make five piles with pairs of shoes. Materials do not have to be costly. A bag of beans or pasta can be purchased at the store and used for counting, adding, and subtracting. Teachers can always have fun making materials with their student as well. Numbers can be made out of construction paper or cardboard and then painted. Teachers can photocopy the following page on hard stock paper and have the students decorate the numbers. Instead of buying expensive tangrams, children can make their own from the pattern on page 55. Also, students can use hundreds charts like the one on page 56 to practice counting and to look for number patterns.

> Many dyslexic children are kinesthetic learners and cannot visualize the mathematical concepts.

Concluding Remarks

Regardless of how math is taught, the dyslexic child may need to have certain skills reinforced while still having the chance to make meaning with the concepts. The dyslexic child may have difficulty reading the math word problem but once he or she understands its meaning might have no difficulty solving the problem. In addition, other subjects such as science and social studies may be areas where the dyslexic child experiences frustration with the reading and writing activities. Children with dyslexia need to be surrounded with exciting activities and encouraged to use their strengths to compensate for their weaknesses.

Numbers to Color

Color these numbers in an interesting way.
Cut them out and use them to make your
own counting book.

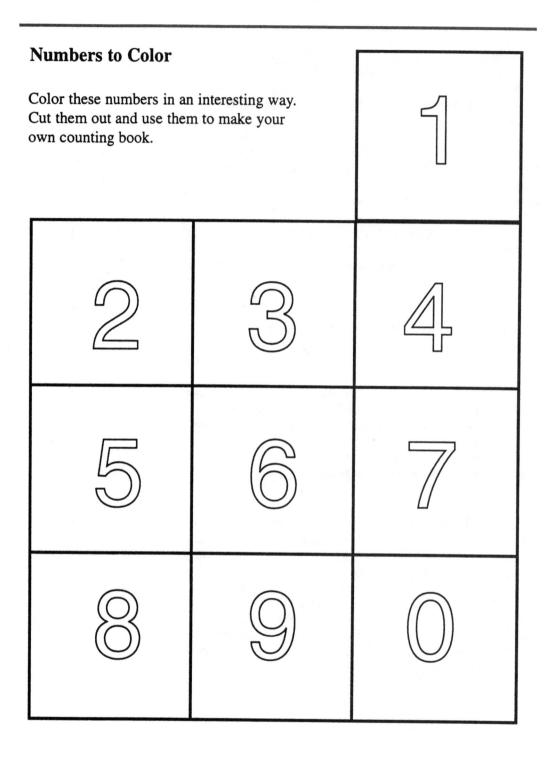

Tangram

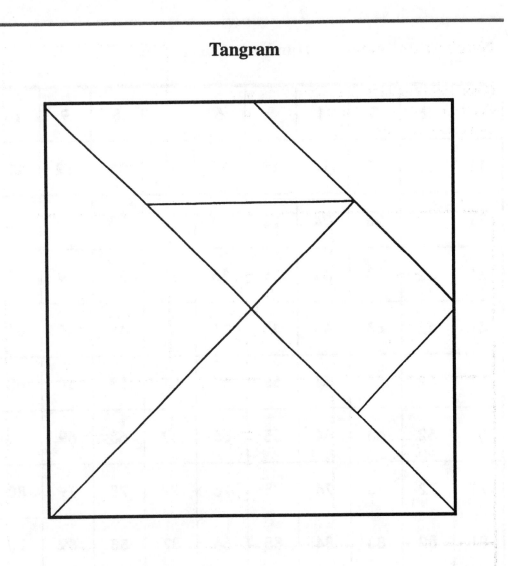

Hundreds Chart

1	2	3	4	5	6	7	8	9	10
11	12	13	14	15	16	17	18	19	20
21	22	23	24	25	26	27	28	29	30
31	32	33	34	35	36	37	38	39	40
41	42	43	44	45	46	47	48	49	50
51	52	53	54	55	56	57	58	59	60
61	62	63	64	65	66	67	68	69	70
71	72	73	74	75	76	77	78	79	80
81	82	83	84	85	86	87	88	89	90
91	92	93	94	95	96	97	98	99	100

Reprinted from TCM Workshop Notebook Hands–On Math, *Teacher Created Materials, 1993*

Methods for Group Work

Group Work

Group work is when small groups of four to five students in the classroom work on the same activity, with each student participating. The goal is for the group to reach a common outcome. Group work is beneficial for the dyslexic child because it increases the time the student is "on task" and actively engaged. Group work can be used in all subject areas and all grade levels. Social interaction among students is natural and group work exposes students to a wide range of opinions and ideas (Bayer, 1990). There are two ways that students can be grouped in the classroom: homogeneously or heterogeneously.

Group work is beneficial for the dyslexic child because it increases the time the student is "on task" and actively engaged.

Homogeneous Grouping

Homogeneous grouping is when students are grouped according to similar academic ability. When students are grouped homogeneously, teachers can easily prepare the material because the students are working at the same level. Many educators believe that students need to be grouped with classmates who are academically similar in order for more learning to take place (Clay, 1979; Dooley, 1993).

However, grouping dyslexic children according to their academic ability can put them in groups below their actual intelligence. In a low reading group, dyslexic students have fewer opportunities for differentiated reading instruction since more time is often spent on decoding skills and less time on comprehension (Cunningham, Hall, & Defee, 1991). Furthermore, students are frequently asked more factual questions rather than interpretive, applicative and transactive questions which foster higher levels of thinking. Another point to consider is that homogeneous grouping in the classroom labels children according to their ability. This lowers the self-esteem of the otherwise bright and capable dyslexic child who is placed in the low ability group (Weinstein, 1984).

Heterogeneous Grouping

Heterogeneous grouping is when students of all ability levels are put in small groups where every member can participate in the same activity. Heterogeneous grouping allows all students to be challenged and accommodated since students of different abilities work together, use each other's strengths, and reach one group outcome (Cohen, 1986). Members of a group with diverse abilities can offer an expanded range of alternative viewpoints which can be used for problem solving activities and intellectual development.

Many believe that dyslexic students cannot learn in heterogeneous groups, fearing they cannot keep up. But, in heterogeneous grouping, the expert or more knowledgeable peer can direct the dyslexic student (Grisham & Molinelli, 1995; Cohen, 1986; Bayer, 1990). A more knowledgeable child guides the dyslexic child through the activity. Gradually, the two begin to share the problem solving functions with the novice taking on the initiative and the expert guiding when the novice falters (Bayer, 1990). When working in reading groups, the child with a better reading ability can guide the dyslexic child and to some extent, tutor the child. The better reader also benefits from being a tutor since he or she is reinforcing skills and boosting self-esteem. A child with dyslexia might be more motivated to learn when working with a high ability student. Dyslexic students benefit from heterogeneous group work since they participate in challenging problem solving activities, watch how other students tackle problems, and feel successful contributing to the group outcome.

Selecting the Groups

If the teacher decides to use heterogeneous grouping, it is important that the teacher take some time to select the students for each group. Each group can have a high achiever, two competent achievers, and a low achiever. The following page can be used when selecting groups.

Selecting Cooperative Groups

Legend
> **HA:** High Achiever
> **SN:** Special Needs Student
> **ESL:** English as a Second Language Student
> **CA:** Competent Achiever

Group One *(example)*	Group Two	Group Three
(HA)	( )	( )
(CA)	( )	( )
(CA)	( )	( )
(SN)	( )	( )
(ESL)	( )	( )
Notes : _____	Notes: _____	Notes: _____
_____	_____	_____

Group Four	Group Five	Group Six
( )	( )	( )
( )	( )	( )
( )	( )	( )
( )	( )	( )
( )	( )	( )
Notes: _____	Notes: _____	Notes: _____
_____	_____	_____

Reprinted from TCM650 Cooperative Learning Activities for Language Arts, *Teacher Created Materials, 1994*

Groups should be no larger than five students so that every member can participate (Cohen, 1986). One way of grouping students is to use roles. Each group has five roles and then a student is selected for each role. For example, five roles in group work can be:

◆ 1. *Facilitator:* sees to it that everyone gets the help he or she needs and is responsible for seeking answers within the group rather than through the teacher.

◆ 2. *Checker:* makes sure that everyone has finished his or her work and answered all the questions.

◆ 3. *Setter:* sets up all the materials so that each child has easy access.

◆ 4. *Cleaner:* puts away all the materials properly and cleans up the work place.

◆ 5. *Reporter:* tells what the group found out during wrapup to the rest of the class.

Of course the teacher may add or change the roles according to the students' needs and the activity at hand. In addition, the students can take on different roles during a larger project so that all the students have a chance to be the facilitator, checker, setter, cleaner, and reporter.

Training the Groups

Before students begin group work, they need to be trained on how to work well with other students. Certain exercises and games that reinforce the principles of group work can be role modeled and played out. An excellent resource from the Community Board of Education is called "Conflict Resolution and Elementary Curriculum" (1990). Activities on cooperation, active listening, communication, and acceptance of divergent points of view are used to explicitly teach children how to work with each other. Students with dyslexia will benefit from lessons on active listening and communication since these are often areas of difficulty.

Rules for the Groups

The rules on the following page should be discussed before the activity and reinforced throughout. These rules coincide with the group work training and focus on taking turns, listening, voting, and working through problems. Group work sets up an environment where all students interact in a positive manner. The child with dyslexia will shine since dyslexics are sometimes better oral communicators than written communicators. Rules should be posted in the classroom so the teacher and students can refer to them at any time.

How We Work Together

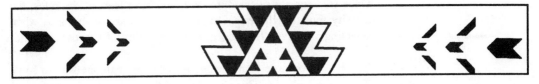

1. When we work in groups, we always take turns.

2. We listen when other people talk.

3. Everyone in the group gets to have a turn.

4. If we cannot agree on something, we vote.

5. If we have a problem, we try to work it out. We do not fight.

6. If we do not know what to do or we have a question, we ask the group first and then the teacher.

Reprinted from TCM650 Cooperative Learning Activities for Language Arts, *Teacher Created Materials, 1994*

Creating an Activity

Once students are selected, trained, and have learned the rules, the activity must be chosen. Certain guidelines should be used when selecting an activity for heterogeneous grouping. The activity should:

◆ 1. have more than one answer or more than one way to solve the problem. This will allow all the students a chance to give solutions and show that there is not just one way to solve a problem.

◆ 2. be intrinsically interesting and rewarding so that all children can be challenged.

◆ 3. have different roles so that all students can contribute.

◆ 4. involve sight, sound, and touch since the dyslexic child and other students might learn better using different senses.

◆ 5. require a variety of skills and behaviors so that all students can participate.

◆ 6. require writing so that each student's thought process in solving the problem is recorded.

At first it may seem overwhelming to come up with a task that follows all these guidelines, but the teacher can monitor and adjust all sorts of activities for group work.

Suggested Activities

Carratello & Carratello (1991) discuss an example of an activity which can be used for heterogeneous group work. In this activity, students work in groups of four to design a world where gentle creatures can be happy. Before the activity, the teacher can brainstorm with the class on what makes people and animals happy. Groups should be encouraged to discuss topics such as geography, economics, and government when creating their world. In addition, the groups can use materials such as construction paper and paint to illustrate their world. This activity is located on page 63.

During the activity, the teacher can give feedback, redirect groups with questions, encourage groups to solve their own problems, and manage conflict (Cohen, 1986). Students with dyslexia might feel more comfortable asking someone in their group a question rather than the teacher. While individual competition is natural, teachers should encourage group success. Group competition can be used as a motivator. I used a point system in group work where teams are rewarded if all members participate, no members fight, and everyone cooperates. Points can be given for teamwork and following rules.

Involve sight, sound, and touch since the dyslexic child and other students might learn better using different senses.

A World for Wumps
and Other Gentle Ones

Would you be able to design a world where Wumps and other gentle creatures could be happy? Work in small groups to plan your new world.

Here are some ideas to help you get started:

• Create a name for your world.

• Decide who will be allowed to live in this world. Be sure to support your inhabitant choices.

• Design a questionnaire that can be used to determine an applicant's worthiness for citizenship.

• Establish rules of conduct that will be required of all inhabitants.

• Make a flag that will be a powerful symbol for your world. Create a motto and creed, too.

• Write a national anthem that will serve to inspire the inhabitants to help your new world stay beautiful.

• Develop an illustrated list of the types of plants that would grow in your world.

• Design living quarters for the inhabitants.

• Plan a system of defense in case others who were not suitable invaded your world.

• Create a brochure to advertise the beauty and harmony of your world.

• Formulate an idea list that would help define your world.

• Write a speech convincing the Wumps to come to your new world.

• Think of more ideas as a group!

Activity to be used with *The Wump World* by Bill Peet (Houghton Mifflin, 1970)

Reprinted from TCM354 Literature Activities for Reluctant Readers, *Teacher Created Materials, 1991*

Evaluating and Grading

Finally, whether the group work was one class period or two weeks, an evaluation should take place so the students can assess the activity, their group performance, and individual performance. First, students can write about the activity, what they liked and did not like, how they might have done it differently, and what they learned. Second, students can reflect on how well they worked in the group and how the group came to a consensus. Third, each student should reflect on his or her own performance and discuss areas of improvement.

When the teacher grades the group work, it is helpful to make observations throughout the activity. Teachers should make notes throughout the activity on student performance and interaction. In addition, each student should receive a group grade and an individual grade. This is important especially for the dyslexic child since many times individual achievement might be low, but when working orally in the group, achievement is high.

Group Process Evaluation

Name _____

Date _____

Members of Your Group _____

_____

Cooperative Task _____

_____

1. Describe the effectiveness of your group on the task.

_____

_____

2. What were the group's strengths?

_____

_____

3. What frustrations did the group encounter?

_____

_____

4. Name one way in which your group could improve in order to be more effective on your next cooperative task.

_____

_____

Reprinted from TCM776 Social Studies Assessment, *Teacher Created Materials, 1994*

Concluding Remarks

If students are properly trained and prepared, then heterogeneous grouping can be the solution to having a classroom with one teacher, thirty students, and little time to reach every child. Everyone, even the dyslexic student, is exposed to grade level curriculum and sometimes more challenging material. When a positive community environment is established, students of different abilities interact and help each other through the activity. The dyslexic student learns to use other students as resources and trust them for support. Finally, the teacher many times can assess a dyslexic child's abilities and special qualities through observation of this interaction.

Assessment in
the Classroom

Problems with Standardized Testing

Many educators feel it is important to assess the knowledge a child has learned by using standardized tests. However, many dyslexic students experience frustration when taking standardized tests. While the dyslexic child often has average or sometimes high intelligence, he or she can receive below average results on standardized tests. Why does this happen? The main reason is that the makeup of the tests may require too much decoding time with little time left for comprehending. In a timed test environment, the dyslexic child may take too long to read and, therefore, not have enough time to answer the questions correctly.

> While the dyslexic child often has average or sometimes high intelligence, he or she can receive below average results on standardized tests.

Authentic Assessment

Assessment in the classroom is the act of making an evaluation of what a child has learned. Educators are seeing a need to move from previous ways of assessing with standardized tests, multiple choice tests, and basal tests toward authentic assessment. Authentic assessment is the process of evaluating the child's performance by gathering evidence and documenting a student's learning and growth in an authentic context (Ryan, 1994). Authentic assessment is extremely beneficial for the child with dyslexia since the assessment is done in an authentic context and not timed. The focus lies on the child's growth, not his or her failure. In addition, the teacher has more freedom to adapt the assessment to the composition of the class and the tendencies of the individual students. The student's strengths are also noted instead of just recording weaknesses, failures, and scores that are compared to other children's scores.

There are many methods of authentically assessing what children know and how much they have learned. In the classroom, the teacher needs to discover the conditions under which a child will perform to his or her best ability. If a dyslexic child is showing a lack of growth, then the teacher may need to assess the conditions under which the child will learn and possibly change instructional methods accordingly.

> The dyslexic child is more motivated to write since he or she is more involved in the assessment process.

Portfolios for Writing

One area where authentic assessment can be of benefit is in the area of writing. Through the use of portfolios, teachers can gather the student's work and have the student reflect on areas of success and areas of growth. The student selects a story that he or she has written and then writes why he or she chose that story for the portfolio. The student then compares this writing to previous work rather than to other students' work. This allows the student to see his or her own growth. The dyslexic child is more motivated to write since he or she is more involved in the assessment process. In assessing the child, the teacher can keep track of the portfolio content and analyze the student's progress.

Assessment for Reading

In order for a teacher to properly assess reading she or he should provide abundant opportunities to read (Vacca, Vacca, & Gove, 1991). Using an interest inventory, teachers can select books that a dyslexic child might be more motivated to read. An interest inventory asks the students questions like: What do you like to do in your free time? What is your favorite sport? and What is your favorite animal? (Ryan, 1994). A sample interest inventory is located on page 71. Teachers can then check out books on these topics and ask students to check them out as well.

Teachers must be good listeners and observers in order to make instructional decisions for the child. A useful way of taking notes and making observations is by using "anecdotal records and observations." Anecdotal records and observations provide a record of an ongoing story about the student's growth and progress (Ryan, 1994). This method is useful when teaching dyslexic students since the teacher is aware of behavioral changes and progress with reading and writing. Teachers can also take into account parent comments and reading at home. A basic anecdotal record form is located on page 72.

Directed Listening-Thinking Activity

The purpose of a directed listening-thinking activity is to assess the child's sense of story structure. Rather then give the student a grammar test, the teacher can authentically assess the student's knowledge of story structure. It is important to be aware of the dyslexic student's knowledge of story structure since children with a sense of story can make the most out of the information that the story presents (Gillet & Temple, 1990). In this assessment, the teacher reads the story aloud to either an individual or small group and pauses several times to ask the students about the characters, setting, or plot. In addition, the teacher can ask the students to predict or hypothesize about what might be most likely to occur next in the story. All responses should be accepted and the environment should be friendly and nonthreatening. Teachers can later record or make note of how the dyslexic student did during the activity. Periodically, the teacher can tape the activity to accurately evaluate the child's performance.

For a teacher, assessment can be used to adjust teaching instruction.

Concluding Remarks

Before a teacher assesses a child, the teacher needs to look at the purpose of assessment and goals. In the classroom, the teacher needs to discover the conditions under which a child will perform to his or her best ability. Using portfolios in the classroom can allow the teacher to observe the growth of each student while giving the students the opportunity to evaluate their own work. It is essential for the dyslexic child to be evaluated according to multiple indicators of student performance (Vacca, Vacca, & Gove, 1991). Teachers should never rely on one test or one observation. It is important to look for patterns and continuity. Many children display dyslexic patterns in their reading and writing which may by transient. The child who needs remediation is the child who displays these patterns regularly and consistently. Authentic assessment allows a teacher with a dyslexic student to truly observe and record what the child does, what learning strategies are being used, and what growth is made.

Overall, the most important thing to remember when working with a child with dyslexia is to never underestimate what the child can do.

Children with dyslexia are usually capable learners who need to be in a supportive and inspiring learning environment. Focus should not be on labeling the child but rather on helping the child use his or her strengths to overcome weaknesses.

Interest Inventory

Student's Name _____ Grade _____

Interviewer _____ Date _____

1. What is your favorite subject in school?

   _____

2. What is your least favorite subject in school?

   _____

3. What do you like to do in your free time?

   _____

4. Who is your best friend?

   _____

5. What is your favorite sport?

   _____

6. What is your favorite animal?

   _____

7. Name something you do very well.

   _____

8. Name something that makes you angry.

   _____

9. What is your favorite TV show?

   _____

10. What is your favorite book?

    _____

11. What is your favorite movie?

    _____

12. If you could meet a famous person, who would it be?

    _____

13. Why would you like to meet that person?

    _____

14. What would you like to learn in school this year?

    _____

Reprinted from TCM777 Language Arts Assessment, *Teacher Created Materials, 1994*

Anecdotal Record Form

Student's Name _____

Date	Observation	Watch for:

Reprinted from TCM777 Language Arts Assessment, *Teacher Created Materials, 1994*

References

Bayer, A. S. (1990). <u>Collaborative-apprenticeship learning</u>. Mountain View, CA: Mayfield Publishing.

Bergman, J. L. (1992). SAIL-A way to success and independence for low-achieving readers. <u>The Reading Teacher, 45</u>, 598–602.

Bradley, L. (1991). <u>Rhyme recognition and reading and spelling in young children. Intimacy with Language</u>. Towson, MD: Orton Dyslexia Society.

Cameron, M., Depree, H., & Walker, J. (1992). <u>Paired-writing: A handbook for teachers</u>. Portsmouth, NH: Heinemann.

Carratello, J., & Carratello, P. (1991). <u>Literature activities for reluctant readers</u>. Westminster, CA: Teacher Created Materials.

Clark, D. B. (1988). <u>Dyslexia: Theory and practice of remedial instruction</u>. Parkton, MD: York Press.

Clay, M. (1979). <u>The early detection of reading differences</u>. Portsmouth, NH: Heinemann.

Cohen, E. (1986). <u>Designing groupwork: Strategies for the heterogeneous classroom</u>. New York: Teachers College Press.

Commeyras, M. (1993). Promoting critical thinking through dialogical-thinking reading lessons. <u>The Reading Teacher, 46</u>, 486–494.

Community Board of Education. (1990). <u>Conflict resolution and elementary curriculum</u>. San Francisco: Author.

Cronin, E. (1994). <u>Helping your dyslexic child</u>. Rocklin, CA: Prima Publications.

Cunningham, P. M., Hall, D., & Defee, M. (1991). Non-ability-grouped, multilevel instruction: A year in a first grade classroom. <u>The Reading Teacher, 44</u>, 566–571.

Depree, H., & Iversen, S. (1993). <u>Wonder world teacher guide: A balanced language program</u>. Bothell, WA: The Wright Group.

Dooley, C. (1993). The challenge: Meeting the needs of gifted readers. <u>The Reading Teacher, 46</u>, 546–551.

Ekwall, E., & Shanker, J. L. (1983). <u>Diagnosis and remediation of the disabled reader</u>, (2nd ed.). Newton, MA: Allyn and Bacon, Inc.

Flowers, D. L. (1993). Brain basis for dyslexia: A summary of work in progress. <u>Journal of Learning Disabilities</u>, 26, 575-582.

Gaskins, R. (1992). Good instruction is not enough: A mentor program. <u>The Reading Teacher, 45</u>, 568–572.

Genishi, C. (1988). Children's language: Learning words from experience. <u>Young Children</u>, 16–23.

Gillet, J., & Temple, C. (1990). <u>Understanding reading problems: Assessment and instruction</u>. New York: HarperCollins.

Graves, D. (1983). <u>Writing: Teachers and children at work</u>. Portsmouth, NH: Heinemann.

Griffith, P., & Olson, M. (1992). Phonemic awareness helps beginning readers break the code. <u>The Reading Teacher, 45</u>, 516–523.

Griffiths, A. (1978). <u>Teaching the dyslexic child</u>. Novato, CA: Academic Therapy Publications.

References *(cont.)*

Grisham, D. L., & Molinelli, P. M. (1995). Cooperative Learning. Westminster, CA: Teacher Created Materials.

Hartwig, L. (1984). Living with dyslexia: One parent's experience. Annals of Dyslexia, 34, 313–317.

Heymsfeld, C. (1992). The remedial child in the whole-language, cooperative classroom. Reading and Writing Quarterly: Overcoming Learning Difficulties, 8, 257–273.

Hinshelwood, J. (1917). Congenital word blindness. London: H.K. Lewis.

Holdaway, D. (1982). Shared book experience: Teaching reading using favorite books. Theory into Practice, 23, 293–300.

Huston, A. (1992). Understanding dyslexia. Lanham, MD: Madison Books.

Johnson, T. D., & Louis, D. R. (1990). Bringing it all together: A program for literacy. Portsmouth, NH: Heinemann.

Jones, R. (1992, September). New theories about dyslexia. American Health, 65–69.

Kamhi, A. (1992). Response to historical perspective: A developmental language perspective. Journal of Learning Disabilities, 25, 48–52.

Labbo, L., & Teale, W. (1990). Cross-age reading: A strategy for helping poor readers. The Reading Teacher, 362-369.

Leslie, L., & Caldwell, J. (1990). Qualitative reading inventory. New York: HarperCollins.

Lyytinen, P., Rasku-Puttonen, H., Poikkeus, A., Laakso, M., & Ahonen, T. (1994). Mother-child teaching strategies and learning disabilities. Journal of Learning Disabilities, 27, 186–192.

Maria, K. (1987). A new look at comprehension instruction for disabled readers. Annals of Dyslexia, 37, 264–278.

Mayo Clinic. (1993). Family Health Book. Eagan, MN: IVI Publishing, Inc.

Meyerson, M. J., & Van Vactor, J. C. (1992). Reading theoretical orientation of teachers who instruct special needs students. Reading Psychology: An International Quarterly, 13, 201–215.

Moffett, J., & Wagner, B. (1992). Student-centered language arts, K–12. Portsmouth, NH: Heinemann.

O'Dell, S. (1960). Island of the blue dolphins. New York: Dell.

Orton, S. (1928). Specific reading disability-strephosymbolia. Journal of American Medical Association, 90.

Orton, S. (1937). Reading, writing, and speech problems in children. New York: Norton.

Rayner, K., & Pollatsek, A. (1989). The psychology of reading. Englewood Cliffs, NJ: Prentice Hall.

Richardson, S. (1989). Specific developmental dyslexia: Retrospective and prospective views. Annals of Dyslexia, 39, 3–23.

Richardson, S. (1992). Historical perspectives on dyslexia. Journal of Learning Disabilities, 25, 40–47.

References *(cont.)*

Routman, R. (1988). <u>Transitions: From literature to literacy</u>. Portsmouth, NH: Heinemann.

Ruddell, R. B. (In Press). <u>Trends and issues in reading instruction</u>. Needham, MA: Allyn and Bacon, Inc.

Ryan, C. (1994). <u>Language arts assessment, Grades 3–4</u>. Westminster, CA: Teacher Created Materials.

Steeves, J. (1979). Make math multi-sensory. <u>Perspectives on Dyslexia, 4</u>, 1-2.

Tierney, R. J., Readence, J., & Dishner, E. (1990). <u>Reading strategies and practices</u>. Needham, MA: Allyn and Bacon, Inc..

Tuttle, C., & Paquette, P. (1994). The learning disabled child and the home. <u>Their World</u>, 91–93.

Vacca, J. L., Vacca, R. T., & Gove, M. (1991). <u>Reading and learning to read</u>. New York: HarperCollins.

Vygotsky, L. S. (1962). <u>Thought and language</u>. Cambridge, MA: MIT Press.

<u>Webster's Ninth New Collegiate Dictionary</u>. (9th ed.). (1987). Springfield, MA: Webster.

Welch, M. (1992). The PLEASE strategy: A metacognitive learning strategy for improving the paragraph writing of students with mild learning disabilities. <u>Learning Disability Quarterly, 15</u>, 119–122.

Weinstein, R. (1984). <u>The teaching of reading and children's awareness of teacher expectations</u>. Paper presented at The Contexts of Literacy Conference, Utah.

Teacher Created Materials
Reference List

TCM #354 Literature Activities for Reluctant Readers
TCM #342 Connecting Math and Literature
TCM #650 Cooperative Learning Activities for Language Arts
TCM #777 Language Arts Assessment, Grades 3-4
TCM #776 Social Studies Assessment, Grades 3-4

TCM Workshop Notebook "Hands–On Math"

Professional Organizations

The Orton Dyslexia Society
Chester Building, Suite 382
8600 La Salle Road
Baltimore, Maryland 21286-2044
(410) 296 - 0232

Slingerland Institute, One Bellevue Center
411 108th Ave. Northeast 230
Bellevue, WA 98004
(206) 453-1190

Parents' Educational Resource Center
1660 South Amphlett Blvd., Suite 200
San Mateo, CA 94402
(415) 513-0920

Lindamood-Bell Learning Process
416 Higuera
San Luis Obispo, CA 93401
(800) 234 - 62248600

Herman Method Institute
4700 Tyrone
Sherman Oaks, CA 91423
(818) 784-9566